LASER DYES

Properties of Organic Compounds for Dye Lasers

LASER DYES

*Properties of Organic Compounds
for Dye Lasers*

MITSUO MAEDA

Department of Electrical Engineering
Kyushu University
Fukuoka, Japan

1984

ACADEMIC PRESS, INC.

(Harcourt Brace Jovanovich, Publishers)

Tokyo   Orlando   San Diego   New York
London   Toronto   Montreal   Sydney

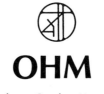

OHM

Tokyo•Osaka•Kyoto

Copublished by
OHMSHA, LTD.
1-3 Kanda Nishiki-cho, Chiyoda-ku, Tokyo 101
and

ACADEMIC PRESS JAPAN, INC.
Hokoku Bldg. 3-11-13, Iidabashi, Chiyoda-ku, Tokyo 102

United States Edition published by ACADEMIC PRESS, INC.
Orlando, Florida 32887

United Kingdom Edition published by ACADEMIC PRESS, INC. (LONDON) LTD.
24/28 Oval Road, London NW1 7DX

Distributed in Japan by Ohmsha, Ltd., and Academic Press Japan, Inc.
Distributed outside Japan by Academic Press, Inc.

Library of Congress Cataloging in Publication Data

Maeda, Mitsuo, Date
   Laser dyes.

   Bibliography: p.
   Includes indexes.
   1. Dye lasers--Materials. I. Title.
TA1690.M33 1984   621.36'64   83-15069
ISBN 0-12-464980-7

PRINTED IN THE UNITED STATES OF AMERICA

84 85 86 87   9 8 7 6 5 4 3 2 1

Contents

Abbreviations

Ac	Acetyl $-COCH_3$
Allyl	$-CH_2CH=CH_2$
Amyl	$-CH_2(CH_2)_3CH_3$
AO filter	Acoust-optic filter
Ar	Argon ion laser
As	Anisyl $-CH_2C_6H_4OCH_3$
ASE	Amplified spontaneous emission
BB	Broad-band operation
BF filter	Birefringent filter
Biphenylyl	$-C_6H_4C_6H_5$
Bu	Butyl $-C_4H_9$
CdS	E-beam pumped CdS semiconductor laser
COT	Cyclooctatetraene
Cu	Copper vapor laser
CW	Continuous wave operation
DFB	Distributed feedback
DMF	N,N-Dimethylformamide
DMSO	Dimethyl sulfoxide
DPA	N,N-Dipropylacetamide
DPB	1,4-Dimethylbutadiene
E	Conversion efficiency
EG	Ethylene glycol
Et	Ethyl $-C_2H_5$
Etalon	Fabry–Perot filter
Excimer	Rare-gas halide excimer laser
FH	Fourth harmonic wave
Fl	Flashlamp pumping
GaAlAs	GaAlAs diode laser
Glass	Neodymium glass laser
HeNe	Helium–neon laser
HFIP	Hexafluoroisopropanol
IF filter	Interference filter
IR	Infrared
i-Pr	Isopropyl $-CH(CH_3)_2$
Kr	Krypton ion laser
MBBA	p-Methoxybenzylidene-p-n-butylaniline

Me	Methyl $-CH_3$
mM	10^{-3} mol/liter
N$_2$	Nitrogen laser
N$_2{}^+$	Nitrogen ion laser
Nd	Neodymium laser (YAG or glass laser)
NP-10	Nonylphenyl substituted by 10 mol of ethylenoxide
OAc	Acetoxy $-OCOCH_3$
Osc + Amp	Oscillator plus amplifier system
Ph	Phenyl $-C_6H_5$
Piperidinyl	$-N\overset{\displaystyle\frown}{\underset{\displaystyle\smile}{}}$
PMMA	Polymethylmethacrylate
Pr	Propyl $-CH_2CH_2CH_3$
PVA	Poly(vinyl acetate)
2-Py	2-Pyridyl $-NC_5H_5$
REB	Relativistic electron beam
RT	Risetime of pumping light
Ruby	Ruby laser
SA	Saturable absorber (saturable dye)
Satur.	Saturated solution
SH	Second harmonic wave
TH	Third harmonic wave
Thr	Input at lasing threshold
Tl	Toly $-C_6H_4CH_3$
Ts	p-Toluenesulfonyl $-SO_3C_6H_4CH_3$
UV	Ultraviolet
W$_{av}$	Average power
W$_{peak}$	Peak Power
YAG	Neodymium yttrium−aluminum−garnet laser

Preface

Organic dye lasers are very useful coherent light sources, which can be tuned over a wide spectral region from ultraviolet to near infrared. Various dye lasers with excellent performance characteristics have been developed and have become powerful tools in various fields of science and engineering. This book is a compilation of organic compounds used for dye lasers.

Since the dye laser was first demonstrated, stimulated emission from many classes of organic compounds has been reported. Although a most detailed list of laser dyes was published by K. H. Drexhage in 1973, many new materials have since been added, and the total number of lasing compounds is now unknown. As a dye laser researcher, I widely surveyed laser dyes in the early stages of development of the field. In the course of this work, I made a set of card files on laser dyes, recording the chemical and lasing data that appeared in various scientific articles. This volume is based on those files. It was first published in *Laser*

Kenkyu (The Review of Laser Engineering) in Japan. The information contained here provides the most comprehensive listing of laser dyes currently available.

For the publication of this book, the text was revised and translated into English. The arrangement of tables and references was changed for the convenience of readers, and misprints were corrected. To avoid confusion, however, the dye and reference code numbers were not changed from the original publication.

I hope that this volume will be widely read, not only by researchers of laser dyes but also by general users of dye lasers. Because accuracy is so important in a publication of this type, I would appreciate being informed of any mistakes or incomplete descriptions.

It is a great pleasure to acknowledge the contributions of many people to the publication of this book. I would like to thank Professor Chiyoe Yamanaka, president of the Laser Society of Japan, and Professor Susumu Namba, chairman of the editorial committee of *Laser Kenkyu,* as well as other members of the editorial committee and office. I must also thank the staff of Nipon Kanko-Shikiso Kenkyusho (Japanese Research Institute for Photosensitizing Dyes Co., Ltd.), Dr. Yasunaga Ogo, the president, and Dr. Ken Banno, Dr. Shigeo Yasui, and Dr. Kenzo Matsutani for their support. I am especially grateful to Dr. Matsutani, who took on the complicated job of dye classification and nomenclature. This proved very helpful to me, inasmuch as I am not a chemist. I also obtained valuable information from the following dye-laser investigators: Professor F. P. Schäfer (Max-Planck Institute), Dr. D. Basting (Lambda Physik), Dr. C. Rulliere (Université de Bordeaux), Dr. K. H. Drexhage (Gesamthochschule Siegen), Drs. Majewski and J. Krasinski (University of Warsaw), Dr. F. B. Dunning (Rice University), and Dr. A. N. Fletcher (United States Navy, Naval Weapons Center). Mr. Yasuya Mutsuura assisted me in making the files, and Mr. Takuji Noguchi was helpful in arranging the lists and preparing the index. Professor Yasushi Miyazoe has continuously supported my research in this field. Finally, I would like to acknowledge all the members of the laser laboratory at Kyushu University.

Mitsuo Maeda

CHAPTER 1

Introduction

The first demonstration of a dye laser was reported in 1966 by Sorokin and Lankard (69), who observed stimulated emission from an alcoholic solution of a phthalocyanine dye pumped by a Q-switched ruby laser. Schäfer et al. (9) and Spaeth and Bortfeld (5) also observed the dye-laser action in cyanine dyes, independently. In 1967, a flashlamp-pumped dye laser was developed (70,75), and both xanthene dyes and coumarin derivatives showed efficient laser action. High-power ultraviolet pulsed lasers, such as N_2 lasers and the higher harmonics of solid-state lasers, were also used for pumping sources to obtain lasing at shorter wavelengths. Various classes of laser dyes have been developed over a wide spectral range from the infrared (IR) to the ultraviolet (UV).

Peterson et al. first demonstrated a continuous-wave (CW) rhodamine 6G dye laser in 1970, using an argon ion laser as a pumping source (106). Excellent performance in coherency and stability was realized by these CW dye lasers. In 1978, an electron-beam-pumped dye vapor laser was reported for POPOP (248).

It is already commonly recognized that dye lasers are one of the most useful and practical of tunable coherent sources. The first experiment of tuning and condensation of the lasing spectrum of a dye laser was made by Soffer and McFarland (273), who placed a

1

Littrow grating inside the dye-laser cavity. The tuning techniques for dye lasers greatly advanced after that; and currently, the spectral width of the frequency-stabilized CW dye laser is as narrow as those of gas lasers. Although the tunable range of each dye is typically 30–50 nm, laser action can be obtained over the entire continuous spectral region from 308.5 to 1285 nm (55,302) by the exchange of dyes. Dye lasers are now contributing greatly to the progress in laser spectroscopy and laser chemistry, and their field of application is rapidly expanding.

Another remarkable feature of dye lasers is the generation of ultra-short pulses. Subpicosecond (10^{-13} s) light pulses are obtained from mode-locked CW dye lasers. This may be the shortest pulse that can be generated in the pulse technology (274). Thus, the dye laser is a pioneer in ultra-high-speed pulse technology.

A wide variety of organic compounds with complex chemical structures is used as the active medium in dye lasers. Many authors have made lists of laser dyes in their reviews (2,60,275,276). The most detailed of them was published by Drexhage (60) with 206 dyes. However, many new materials have been reported since then. This book contains a new compilation of organic compounds usable for dye lasers. The features of this compilation are as follows:

1. All lasing organic chemicals reported up to 1980 are listed. Five hundred forty-six dyes are recorded. Some new references were added in proofreading.
2. The chemical name, chemical structure, trivial name, abbreviated name, trade name, and so on, are recorded as much as possible. Because the chemical name is usually too long, the same substance is sometimes called by a number of different names, which causes confusion.
3. Many examples of published experimental data on the lasing of each dye are listed. Readers will be able to learn a dye's general characteristic from this information, although the performance of each dye usually varies according to experimental conditions.

CHAPTER 2

Classification of Lasing Compounds

Although "dye" means, of course, a colored substance, many uncolored organic fluorescent materials are used for dye lasers. Thus the definition of the dye laser should be as follows: *a laser utilizing an allowed transition of conjugated π electrons in organic molecules.* Typical absorption and fluorescence spectra of several organic compounds for dye lasers are shown in Fig. 1. The longest absorption maximum is due to the transition from the electronic singlet ground state S_0 to the first excited singlet state S_1. When this absorption band is in the visible region, the substance is colored. The band is composed of a continuum of vibrational and rotational levels. No discrete vibrational or rotational level is observed in such complex organic molecules in general.

Fluorescence is due to the allowed transition $S_1 \to S_0$, whose lifetime is on the order of ns. The high fluorescence quantum yield is essential for laser action. The fluorescence band has a typical width of 100 nm on which the tunability of dye lasers depends.

The lasing compounds are divided into classes according to their chemical structures and arranged as such in the compilation. However, this arrangement may be inconvenient for general dye

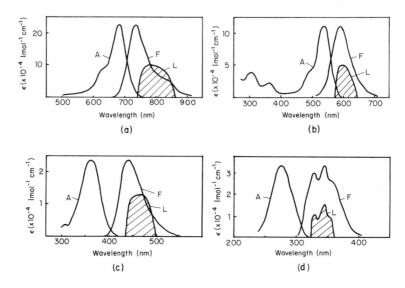

Fig. 1. Absorption (A), fluorescence (F), and typical laser tuning (L) curves for some compounds. (a) #M43 (DOTC) in DMSO, (b) #M94 (rhodamine 6G) in ethanol, (c) #M330 (Coumarin 1) in ethanol, and (d) #M206 (p-terphenyl) in cyclohexane. Vertical axis: (A) molar extinction coefficient $\epsilon(\times 10^{-4}\ \mathrm{lmol^{-1}\ cm^{-1}})$, (F) and (L) arbitrary unit.

laser users who are not chemists. For these people, an alphabetical name index is at the back of this book.

Table 1 lists the general classification of the compounds and the table number in which they are listed. Figure 2 shows the distribution of the lasing wavelengths for some important classes of compounds. The lasing wavelengths in this figure represent the central wavelength of the tunable range in each dye. Each line in this figure corresponds to one compound.

Both chemical name and structure are shown in the compilation. The chemical structures are given at the end of each table to save space. As for the nomenclature, names in common use are shown. Sometimes the formal nomenclature of organic compounds is ignored when it is too long, because most readers are not specialists in organic chemistry. The abbreviated names and trade names that appear often in the literature have been collected

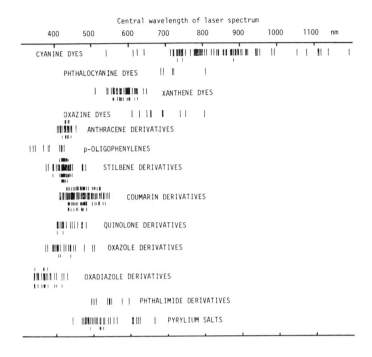

Fig. 2. Distribution of lasing wavelengths of each dye class. Each lasing wavelength in this figure indicates the central wavelength of the widest tunable region in each dye.

as much as possible. A list of chemical structures and various names of 30 famous dyes has been published by Kauffman (277).

Every compound is given a serial code number (#M). Even if the chemical structure is slightly different, they are considered different materials; however, if the difference is only in anions, for example, perchlorate (ClO_4^-), chloride (Cl^-), bromide (Br^-), iodide (I^-), they are considered to be the same material.

The data shown in the first line of the compilation represents the first report published on each dye. Below that, however, the data are not always arranged in the order of publication. There is a great deal of literature on dye lasers and their applications. Although it is impossible to investigate all this literature, I endeavored to quote useful data whenever possible. As for several popular dyes, such as rhodamine 6G, only typical experiments are shown. The investigated literature is limited to scientific publication. However, information obtained from something like catalogs or data sheets, distributed by manufacturers of dye lasers and chemicals, are also recorded if they are useful.

Table 1.   General Classification and Table Index

Classification	Table no.	Dye no.
I. Dyes		
Cyanine		
Carbocyanine	4	#M1 - #M9
Dicarbocyanine	5	#M10 - #M28
Tricarbocyanine	6	#M29 - #M65
Tetracarbocyanine	7	#M66 - #M68
Pentacarbocyanine	8	#M69 - #M73
Merocyanine	10	#M74 - #M78
Phthalocyanine	11	#M79 - #M83
Xanthene	12	#M84 - #M122
(including rhodamine and fluorescein)		
Triarylmethane	13	#M123-#M127
Acridine	14	#M128-#M134
Azine	15	#M135-#M149
(including oxazine and thiazine)		
Chlorophylls	16	#M150-#M154
Miscellaneous	17	#M155-#M167
II. Aromatic compounds		
Condensed ring	18	#M168-#M205
(include naphthalene, anthrathen, pylene, and perylene)		
Ologophenylenes	19	#M206-#M215
(included p-terphenyl and p-quaterphenyl)		

(continued)

Table 1 *(continued)*

	Classification	Table no.	Dye no.
	Conjugated diene	20 and 21	#M216-#M268
	Miscellaneous	22	#M271-#M272
III.	Heterocyclic compounds		
	Coumarin derivatives (included azacoumarin)	23 and 24	#M277-#M380, #M542-#M546
	Quinolone derivatives (included azaquinolone)	25	#M381-#M410
	Oxazole derivatives	26 and 27	#M411-#M438
	Oxadiazole derivatives	28	#M439-#M471
	Furan derivatives	29	#M472-#M473
	Pyrazoline derivatives	30	#M474-#M477
	Phthalimide derivatives (included naphthalimide)	31	#M478-#M486
	Pteridine derivatives	32	#M487-#M490
	Heterocyclic salts (included pyrylium, thiapyrylium, phosphorine, and pyridine salts)	33 and 34	#M491-#M536
	Miscellaneous	35	#M537-#M541

CHAPTER 3

General Remarks on the Tables

I. Excitation Sources

Every dye laser is operated by optical pumping, except for one that is operated by electron beam pumping (278). There are two types of light sources used for optical pumping, that is, coherent and incoherent sources. CW operation is attained only for coherent sources. In Table 2, various excitation sources used for dye lasers are listed.

Flashlamps for dye lasers are usually designed to have much shorter risetimes than those of solid-state lasers, typically 100–500 ns. Because of triplet-state absorption (102), most of the dyes cannot lase in slow pumping. Two types of flashlamps, the linear and coaxial type (102,279), are widely used and commercially available. Xenon is the usual filling gas. In the wall-abrasion-type flashlamp (280,281), the discharge tube is always evacuated down to 1 Torr and the discharge maintained in abraded gas from the tube wall. The voltex-flow-type flashlamp is also useful for its high repetition rate (112,282). Incoherent radiation from a pulsed-CO_2 laser-produced plasma is usable for pumping (115,187).

Short-pulse lasers in the visible or UV region are efficient pumping sources of dye lasers over a wide spectral region. Because the risetime of these laser emissions is 10 ns or so, triplet

absorption can usually be ignored. Therefore, the correlation be-
tween the fluorescence quantum yield and laser efficiency is large
in this type of pumping. As the single-pass gain is very large, a
strong amplified spontaneous emission (ASE) is often observed.

A YAG laser and its higher harmonics are attractive pumping
sources. High-power and efficient lasing are promised over the
largest tunable range. The N_2 laser is a convenient and economic
pumping source with a high repetition rate (up to 100 Hz). Recently developed rare-gas halide excimer lasers show efficient ($\sim$
2%), high-power (>10 MW) laser action in UV (283). The XeCl
laser (lasing wavelength 308 nm) is the most suitable pumping
source for dye lasers. Because the absorption band of dye molecules spreads toward shorter wavelengths, laser action even in IR
as well as in UV and visible regions can be obtained by UV-laser
pumping. The advantage of the Cu vapor laser lies in its high
efficiency, high average power, and high repetition frequency
(several kHz).

Continuous wave operation is realized with an argon or krypton
ion laser. Strong visible lines from blue to green in an argon laser
are most useful. Because the lasing lines of the krypton laser are
distributed over a wide spectral region from UV to IR, it is suitable
for wide wavelength range operation. Frequency stabilized single-
mode (transverse and axial) operation is possible in these CW dye
lasers.

In the "Excitation" column, the name of the excitation source,
strength (power or energy) of the excitation, pump pulse duration
(or risetime, RT), and repetition frequency are listed. The wavelengths and abbreviated symbols of the excitation sources are
given in Table 2. For flashlamp pumping, the electrical energy
charged in the capacitor is indicated.

II. Lasing Wavelength

The lasing wavelength can be varied within the gain bandwidth
(fluorescence bandwidth). When the optical cavity is not wavelength selective, the laser action occurs around its gain maximum

wavelength, and the emission spectrum is broad (3–20 nm). Let us call it *broad-band* (BB) operation. In this case, the lasing wavelength depends on various experimental conditions (284), such as the dye concentration, solvent, additives, temperature, pH, pumping strength, cavity Q value, and cavity length. Therefore, wavelength tuning is possible by changing one of these parameters. This is called *self-tuning*. Self-tuning is predominantly caused by the self-absorption $S_0 \rightarrow S_1$, so that remarkable tuning occurs for molecules whose adsorption and emission bands overlap each other to a great degree.

When a wavelength-selective element is put inside the dye-laser cavity, the lasing spectrum can be externally controlled and narrowed. Typical tuning curves are shown in Fig. 1. Frequency tuners used for dye lasers are listed in Table 3. Dispersion and optical insertion loss are the important points of these tuners, although no substantial loss in spectral condensation exists because of the homogeneous broadening of the fluorescence band.

The dispersion of the diffraction grating is large, but optical loss is also large. A very narrow bandwidth is obtained, especially when the grating is used together with a beam expander (285) or in a grazing incidence configuration (286,287). Because insertion loss is small for the brewster-cut prism or birefringent (BF) filter, they can be used for small-gain lasers such as CW dye lasers. The BF filter is made of a polished crystal plate or its accumulation (Lyot or Solc filter). By the use of an electrooptical crystal, fast electrical tuning of wavelengths is possible. The Fabry–Perot etalon, whose spectral resolution is very high, can be used for fine tuning. A compact and narrow-band dye laser can be constructed by means of the distributed feedback (DFB) configuration (288,289). A sort of diffraction grating is formed in the active medium itself.

The bandwidths of these tunable elements generally depend on the optical beam divergence, and for intense excitation it tends to increase. Adding a dye amplifer is a very effective method of avoiding intense excitation for the oscillator, especially for short-pulse, high-power laser pumping. This scheme is called an *oscillator and amplifier* (Osc + Amp) configuration.

The use of a ring-type optical resonator is also effective for improving spectral quality. Remarkable improvement is reported for single-mode CW dye lasers (84). This effect can be understood in terms of spatial inhomogeneity due to standing waves.

In the column "Lasing wavelength (tuning)," the following items are described. For BB operation the central wavelength of the laser emission is indicated. In the case of self-tuning, the varied parameter is shown, for example, BB concentration or BB cavity length. For external tuning, the broadest tunable wavelength range is given, and the tunable element is shown in parentheses. If various tunable elements are used in cascade, only an important one is shown. The tunable range is not as strict in dye lasers as in other lasers because of their remarkable dependence on experimental conditions. As I sometimes estimated the tunable range from the tuning curves printed in his sources, there may be considerable error.

III. Solvent and Additives

In dye lasers, the dye is mixed or doped in either of the following host materials: (1) an organic or inorganic liquid solvent, (2) a plastic host or organic crystal, (3) a liquid crystal matrix, and (4) buffer gas or vacuum (in vaporized phase).

The ordinal form is the liquid phase. The solvent and its concentration are important factors in determining the lasing wavelength and efficiency. Sometimes two solvents are mixed together. The viscosity is also an important factor in the case of the jet nozzle configuration. The dye concentration is indicated in units of mM (1 mM = 10^{-3} mol/liter) or g/liter in the compilation. The saturated solution is shown by "Satur."

There are four types of additives that can improve lasing performance.

1. Triplet quencher, which suppresses the accumulation of dye molecules in the triplet state. Cyclooctatetraene (COT) is a famous triplet quencher effective in many dyes (74). The oxygen molecules dissolved in the air-saturated solution also

quench the triplet state. *Dioxygenated* means that these oxygen molecules have been removed from the solvent.

2. Surface active agent to prevent the dimerization of dye molecules. Ammonyx LO and Triton X-100 are good additives for aqueous solvents in which fluorescence quenching by dimerization is remarkable (106).

3. Mixing of lasing compounds. When excited energy is successfully transferred from donor molecules to acceptor molecules, the latter are sensitized. In this case, the donor molecules are considered the additive.

4. To control the pH value in the solution, a small amount of NaOH or acid is added. The compilation indicates the pH value.

With vapor-phase dye lasers, the dye is placed in an oven and heated to obtain a suitable vapor pressure. The oven temperature is indicated in this case.

IV. Output

The standardization of the outputs of dye lasers is fairly difficult, as they depend greatly on experimental conditions. For example, the output power is decreased by adding some tuning elements, whereas spectral quality is improved. The output also decreases at wavelengths near the edge of the tuning curve. It should be noted that the compilation shows the "*most efficient result described in the paper concerned.*" If that value is measured in BB operation, energy loss will be inevitable to some extent in the use of a tuner.

The outputs are indicated by power [average power (W_{av}) or peak power (W_{peak})] or total energy with its pulse duration. When such data are not available, this column indicates the conversion efficiency in energy or power, threshold for laser action, and so on. For example, "$E = 10\%$" means "conversion efficiency from input to output is 10%"; "$Thr = 10$ J" means "threshold input energy is 10 J," where input is considered the electric input for flashlamp pumping and optical input for laser pumping.

V. Mode Locking

The mode-locked pulse durations of dye lasers are very short because the gain bandwidth of the dye molecules is large. Light pulses down to 40 fs can be generated by a CW dye laser.

Both passive and active methods can be used for mode locking. In passive mode locking, a saturable absorber (SA) dye is put inside the cavity. Most of the good SAs belong to the cyanine dye group; for example, DODCI is a famous SA for the rhodamine 6G laser.

Active mode locking is obtained by internal modulation. The synchronous pumping method is important for obtaining mode locking in laser-pumped dye lasers (274,290). In synchronous pumping, a mode-locked laser is used as a pumping source. The dye laser is synchronously mode locked by taking equal cavity lengths of the pumping laser and dye laser.

The advantage of active mode locking is that the operation is stable and no wavelength limitation exists. However, the shortest pulses are generated in passive mode locking.

Table 2. Excitation Sources and Their Wavelengths Used for Dye Laser

Source	Wavelength (nm)	Abbreviation
Coherent		
CW (including CW mode locking)		
Argon ion laser	Visible and UV[a]	Ar
Krypton ion laser	IR, visible, and UV[b]	Kr
He-Ne laser	632.8	HeNe
CW dye laser		CW dye
Pulsed		
Nd:glass or Nd:YAG laser	1060	Glass or YAG
Second, third, and fourth harmonics	530, 353, and 265	SH-, TH-, and FH-
Ruby laser and its second harmonics	694.3 and 347.2	Ruby and SH-Ruby
Nitrogen laser	337.1 and IR (1054– 750, 33 lines)	N_2 and IR N_2
Nitrogen ion laser	427.8	N_2^+
Copper vapor laser	510.5 and 578.2	Cu
Rare-gas halide excimer laser		Excimer
XeF, KrF, and XeCl	353, 249, and 308	XeF, KrF, and XeCl

(continued)

Table 2 *(continued)*

Source	Wavelength (nm)	Abbreviation
Semiconductor laser		
GaAlAs diode laser	820	GaAlAs diode
e-beam-pumped CdS laser	494	CdS
Xenon-ion laser	364.5 (and in blue-green)	Xe
Pulsed-dye laser		Pulsed dye
Incoherent		
Flashlamp		Fl
CO_2-laser-produced plasma		CO_2 laser plasma
Relativistic electron beam		REB

[a] Visible (528.7, 514.5*, 501.7, 496.5, 488.0*, 476.5, 472.7, 465.8, 457.9, and 454.5 nm) UV (368.8, 351.4, 351.1, 333.6 nm) (* strong line).

[b] IR (799.3, 793.1, and 752.5 nm). Visible (676.4, 647.1*, 568.2, 530.9, 520.8, 482.5, 476.2, 468.0, 415.4, 413.1, and 406.7 nm) UV (356.4, 350.7, and 337.5 nm) (* strong line).

Table 3. Tuning Elements Used for Dye Lasers

Element	Abbreviation
Diffraction grating	Grating
Prism	Prism
Fabry-Perot etalon	Etalon
Birefringent filter	BF filter
Acoustooptic filter	AO filter
Distributed feedback	DFB
Interference filter	IF filter
Fizeau interferometer wedge	
Farady filter	

CHAPTER 4

Dyes

In this section, the term *dye* is used in its original meaning, namely, *colored substance*. The first dye laser was born in the IR region. The longer wavelength part (>530 nm) of the spectral region is charged by these dyes.

There are several classes of dyes with which laser action has been reported. Most of the important dyes are derivatives of a substituted tricyclic ring. Two classes of dyes with an oxygen bridge in this ring, rhodamine and oxazine dyes, have special importance for dye lasers. On the other hand, cyanine dyes are useful in very long wavelengths and have a unique structure.

I. Cyanine Dyes

Because this class of dye molecules has a long conjugated methine chain (—CH = CH—), the dyes are sometimes called *polymethine dyes*. An important use of these dyes has been the color sensitization of photographic films.

The general formula is shown in Fig. 3, where ϕ and ψ are heterocyclic radicals with a nitrogen bridge, and n is the number of methine radicals. Cyanine dyes have a remarkable nature in

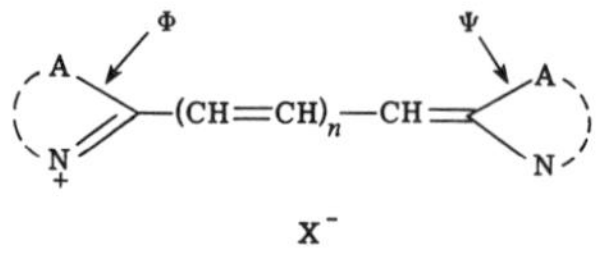

Fig. 3. General structure of cyanine dyes ($n = 0, 1, 2, \ldots$).

that the absorption and fluorescence bands shift to longer wavelengths by $\sim$100 nm and with every one unit increase in n. This
phenomenon can be understood in terms of a simple free-electron
model developed by Kuhn (61). That model provides a good example of a color formation mechanism of substances analyzed by
the behavior of conjugated electrons. As a result, the lasing wavelengths of cyanine dyes are distributed over a wide spectral region, as shown in Fig. 2. Hydrogen atoms in the methine chain are
sometimes substituted.

In the tables the lists are arranged by the length of the methine
chain n as follows: (1) Table 4 *carbocyanine* (#M1–#M9: $n = 1$);
(2) Table 5 *dicarbocyanine* (#M10 − #M28: $n = 2$); (3) Table 6
tricarbocyanine (#M29–#M65: $n = 3$); ($) Table 7 *tetracarbo-
cyanine* (#M66–#M68: $n = 4$); (5) Table 8 *pentacarbocyanine*
(#M69–#M73: $n = 5$). No laser action is observed for the dyes $n = 0$, as they are not fluorescent (291). From a practical viewpoint,
cyanine dyes are useful in the spectral range longer than 800 nm,
where no dye competes with them. The longest lasing wavelength
ever reported is 1285 nm, attained with a pentacarbocyanine dye
(#M70) (55). Theoretically, one could get a dye whose wavelength
is longer than that by extending the methine chain; however, it
would be chemically unstable and could not be used for lasers.

In the early stage of dye-laser research, efficient laser action of
various cyanine dyes pumped by a ruby laser was reported (9,22).
A systematic investigation of this class of dyes was done by me in
that period (3,4). A lot of cyanine dyes have been prepared by
Nippon Kanko-Shikiso Kenkyusho (Japanese Research Institute
for Photosensitizing Dyes Company, Ltd.) (292), and also by Eastman Kodak Company (32,293). Nd:glass and Nd:YAG laser are

good pumping sources for the longest IR region (53,55,58). Operation by flashlamp pumping is also possible. UV pumping with N_2 or excimer laser is possible, although the conversion efficiency is small. Efficient CW operation is obtained by pumping with red and IR lines of the krypton ion laser. The long wavelength limit for CW operation is 1020 nm (49) and for CW mode-locked operation, 1095 nm (46).

Cyanine dye molecules form fluorescent photoisomers during the excitation in general, and their lasing is observed in longer wavelengths (62,63). Dimethyl sulfoxide (DMSO) is a good solvent for this class of dyes in general. For quinocarbocyanines, high efficiency is promised by a viscous solvent such as glycerin.

Some of the cyanine dyes have rather poor chemical stability. They must be kept in a dark and cold place. The life of the solvent is short. Preparation of a fresh sample is required to obtain high efficiency, especially for IR dyes.

About 18 dyes, which are pumpable with a Nd laser, are reported in ref. (51) and (65). However, compilation contains only #M69, because the identification is difficult.

Cyanine dyes are very important materials both as SAs for solid-state lasers and dye lasers, and as a laser medium (274).

II. Merocyanine Dyes

Table 10 lists laser performances and chemical structures of merocyanine dyes. In addition, Danilov (170) and Aristov et al. (171) have reported lasing in several "ketocyanine dyes" pumped by a glass laser (SHG) and flashlamp. These dyes may belong to merocyanine or cyanine dyes, but are unrecorded in the compilation because the details are unknown. The first report on DCM (#M78) is reference 176 (67). DCM (#M78) shows very efficient CW laser action in 610–710 nm (297,303). It is one of the most efficient and stable dyes in this spectral region.

III. Phthalocyanine Dyes

It should be remembered that chloroaluminum phthalocyanine showed the first laser action, as reported by Sorokin and Lankard (69). Phthalocyanine dyes are generally strong with regard to bleaching, and useful as a brilliant blue painting material. However, the lasing performances are inferior to cyanine dyes (Table 11).

IV. Xanthene Dyes

Xanthene dyes have a xanthene ring, shown in Fig. 4a as a chromophore. These beautiful dyes are widely utilized in color cloths, papers, cosmetics, foodstuffs, etc. Xanthene dyes are classified into the following two types: (1) *rhodamine type* (#M84–#M111): the 2- and 7-positions in the xanthene ring are substituted by amino (NH_2) radicals (Fig. 4b) and (2) *fluorescein type* (#M112–#M120): the 2- and 7-positions in the xanthene ring are substituted by hydroxyl (OH) radicals (Fig. 4c).

Rhodamine dyes are the most important group of all laser materials. As is well known, rhodamine 6G (#M94) has been a standard for evaluating other dyes ever since various ways of laser operation were first tried. Drexhage et al. developed new rhodamine dyes to expand the tunable region from green to red (83). For example, a tunable range from 540 to 690 nm can be covered by three dyes, rhodamine 110 (#M88), rhodamine 6G (#M94), and rhodamine 101 (#M109).

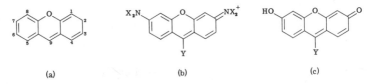

(a)   (b)   (c)

Fig. 4. Structures of (a) xanthene ring, (b) rhodamine type, and (c) fluorescein type.

The lasing efficiency of rhodamine dyes is very high, and the chemical stability fairly good. An energy conversion efficiency of over 50% is available for green pumping sources such as SHG of YAG laser or Cu vapor laser (50,172). The visible laser lines of argon ions are also very effective pumping sources, and an output power of 52 W is obtained at the maximum (117). For flashlamp pumping, the available maximum output is 400 J per pulse (111) and 100 W average power (112,113). These are the largest outputs of all dye lasers ever reported.

Alcohol is the usual solvent for rhodamine dyes. When an aqueous solvent is used, a few *percent* of Ammonyx LO or Triton X-100 should be added. For the jet nozzle configuration (294), ethylene glycol is preferred. A triplet quencher COT is effective in increasing the output to some extent.

The lasing wavelengths of fluorescein dyes are shorter than those of rhodamine dyes, which are typically in the green region. Fluorescein (#M112) emits strong fluorescence in a weak alkali solution. Cyclooctatetraene is also effective in this type of dye; however, the overall efficiency is inferior to those of rhodamine dyes and possibly coumarin dyes, whose lasing wavelengths are in the same spectral region.

The lasing characteristics and chemical structures of xanthene dyes are shown in Table 12. The author assigned serial numbers, rhodamine derivatives 1–12, to many rhodamine dyes investigated by Levin et al. (81) and Neporent et al. (124) for the sake of convenience. As some of their structures are unknown, they are estimated (* represents one that has been estimated). According to the chemical list of Eastman Kodak Company (293), rhodamine 116 and rhodamine 123 are recorded as laser dyes. However, these dyes are not recorded in the compilation because no report on their lasing has been found.

V. Triarylmethane Dyes

Triarylmethane dyes lack the oxygen bridge in the xanthene ring. Their lasing was reported earlier with the excitation of a ruby laser, as shown in Table 13.

VI. Acridine Dyes

Acridine dyes have an acridine ring, shown in Fig. 5 as a chromophore. A typical acridine dye replaces the 2- and 7-positions with amino radicals (#M128 and #M131). Carbazine 122 (#M134) is classified in this group. It should be noted that acridine red (#M84) does not belong to this class (Table 14).

VII. Azine Dyes

One azine dye is historically known as the oldest synthesized dye. Azine dyes have a heterocyclic ring with a nitrogen bridge, as shown in Fig. 6. They can be classified further by the atom X:

1. X = O oxazine dyes   #M135–#M144
2. X = S thiazine dyes   #M145–#M148
3. X = N diazine (phenazine) dyes   #M149

Oxazine dyes are very important materials for dye lasers, especially at longer wavelengths than those of rhodamine dyes (see Table 15). In the IR region, they compete with cyanine dyes, but they are better with regard to chemical stability. Cresyl violet (#M140) is a well-known dye in this class. Some new oxazine dyes have been developed by Eastman Kodak Company (60,83). Laser action over a wavelength range from 640 to 760 nm is possible with a combination of cresyl violet (#M140), nile blue (#M139), and oxazine-1 (#M136). Mixing with a rhodamine dye is effective for short wavelength excitation, because the excitation energy transfer is efficient. Efficient (~30%) CW operation is reported with 647- and 676-nm lines of the krypton laser.

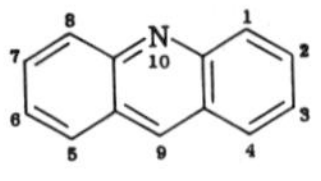

Fig. 5. Structure of acridine ring.

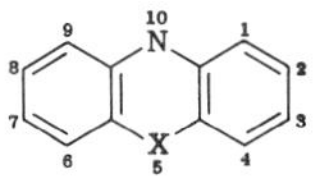

Fig. 6. Structure of azine (X = O, oxazine; X = S, thiazine; X = N, diazine).

VIII. Chlorophylls

It is very interesting that laser action is obtained with natural fluorescent dyes, chlorophylls, as shown in Table 16. Rubinov and Mostovnikov (173) and Mory *et al.* (174) reported on lasing in chlorophylls before Hindman *et al.* (151). However, Table 16 does not include their data, because it is unclear what kind of chlorophyll they used.

IX. Miscellaneous Dyes

Table 17 lists miscellaneous dyes or dyes whose chemical structure is unknown.

LD700 (#M167), developed by Exciton Chemical Company (152), shows very efficient CW laser action in 700-nm region by Kr laser pumping. However, its chemical structure has not been published.

Many new dyes are recorded in the latest catalog of Exciton Chemical Company (152): LD 688, LDS 698 (pyridine 1), LDS 722 (pyradine 2), LDS 730 (styryl 6), LDS 750 (styryl 7), LDS 751 (styryl 8), LDS 765, LDS 798 (styryl 11), LDS 820 (styryl 9), LDS 821, LDS 860 (styryl 10), LDS 867, LDS 930, and LDS 965. Efficient CW laser action of styryl 8, 9, 10, and 11 has been reported in the red and IR regions (315–317). The chemical name of styryl 10 is 2-[6-(p-dimethylaminophenyl-1,3,5-hexatrienyl)-3-ethyl](6,7-benzo)benzothiazolium perchlorate (317).

Table 4. Carbocyanine Dyes and Their Laser Characteristics[a]

Solvent	Concentration (mM)	Lasing wavelength (tuning) (nm)	Excitation	Output	Ref.
#M1 3,3'-Diethylthiacarbocyanine iodide; DTC; NK 76					
Glycerin	0.2	625 (BB)	Fl (9 J, 80 ns, RT)	Thr = 4.6 J	1
#M2 3,3'-Diethyloxacarbocyanine iodide; DOC; NK 85					
Glycerin	0.2	541 (BB)	Fl (9 J, 80 ns, RT)	Thr = 1.3 J	1
#M3 1,3,3,1',3',3'-Hexamethylindocarbocyanine iodide; HIC; NK 79					
Glycerin	0.2	614 (BB)	Fl (9 J, 80 ns, RT)	Thr = 1.6 J	1
#M4 1,1'-Diethyl-2,4'-quinocarbocyanine iodide; dicyanine; NK 138					
Glycerin		756 (BB)	Ruby		2
Isobutanol		765 (BB)	Ruby		
Quinoline		723, 752 (BB)	Ruby		

#M5 1,1'-Dimethyl-4,4'-quinocarbocyanine iodide; NK 14

Glycerin	0.1	749 (BB)	Ruby (20 MW, 18 ns)		3
EG	0.1		Ruby (25 MW, 10-15 ns)	E = 7%	4

#M6 1,1'-Diethyl-4,4'-quinocarbocyanine iodide (bromide, chloride); cryptocyanine; NK 5; NK 36; NK 37

Glycerin	0.1	745 (BB)	Ruby (100 MW)		5
Methanol	$5 \times 10^{16}-10^{17}$ (cm^{-3})	808.5 (BB)	Ruby (0.5 J, 30-40 ns)	E = 10%	6
Glycerin	0.1	751 (BB) 754 (BB) bromide	Ruby (20 MW, 18 ns)		3
EG	0.1	747 (BB) bromide chloride	Ruby (25 MW, 10-15 ns)	E = 12.4% E = 10.3% E = 10.3%	4
Glycerin	0.017	745 (BB)	Ruby (100 MW/cm^2)	E = 13%	7

#M7 1,1'-Di-n-butyl-4,4'-quinocarbocyanine iodide; NK 44

EG	0.1	(BB)	Ruby (25 MW, 10-15 ns)	E = 11.2%	4

(continued)

Table 4 (continued)

Solvent	Concentration (mM)	Lasing wavelength (tuning) (nm)	Excitation	Output	Ref.
	#M8 5,5'-Bis[4-(2-benzothiazolyl)-2-yl]-1,3,1',3'-tetraethyl-benzimidazolocarbocyanine perchlorate				
Alcohol	(BB)		Ruby or glass-SH (30 ns)		8
	#M9 1,3,1',3'-Tetra-2-pyridylbenzimidazolocarbocyanine perchlorate				
Alcohol	(BB)		Ruby or glass-SH (30 ns)		8

[a] Structures (see also Table 9):

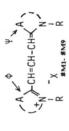

Dye no.	Φ; Ψ	R	X	Dye no.	Φ; Ψ	R	X
#M1	(a)	Et	I	#M6	(t)	Et	I,Br,Cl
#M2	(n)	Et	I	#M7	(t)	n-Bu	I
#M3	(p)	Me	I	#M8	(w)	Et	ClO_4
#M4	(s);(t)	Et	I	#M9	(x)	2-Py	ClO_4
#M5	(t)	Me	I				

Table 5. Dicarbocyanine Dyes and Their Laser Characteristics[a]

Solvent	Concentration (mM)	Lasing wavelength (tuning) (nm)	Excitation	Output	Ref.
#M10 3,3'-Diethylthiadicarbocyanine iodide (perchlorate); DTDC; NK 136; Red 9					
Methanol	0.1	731 (BB)	Ruby (5 MW, 10 ns)		9
Acetone	0.1–0.4	710–730 (BB, concentration)	Ruby (20 MW, 18 ns)		3
DMSO	0.02–0.8	708–743 (BB, concentration	Ruby (25 MW, 10–15 ns)	E = 9.4%	4
DMSO	0.05	754 (BB)	Fl (60 J, 150 ns, RT)	Thr = 34 J (90 ns)	10
DMSO	0.2	759 (BB)	Fl (9 J, 80 ns, RT)	Thr = 2.9 J	1
DMSO	0.2	760 (BB)	Fl (100 J, 100 ns, RT)	Thr = 9.5 J	11
Methanol or EG			Mode-locked HeNe (intracavity pump)		12
Ethanol + rhodamine B	25 + 5	685–740 (prism + grating)	N_2 (130 kW)	2.2 kW	13
+ rhodamine B		670–772 (grating, concentration)	N_2 (250 kW)	>10 kW	14

Water + 1.5% Triton X-100		700–720 (grating)	Ruby (20 MW, 40 ns)		15
DMSO	100	743.5 (grating) 746 (grating) perchlorate	N_2 (100 kW, 10 ns, 100 Hz)		16
Acetone	2	695–725 (grating)	N_2 (300 kW; 10 ns)	0.8–1 ns	17
Glycerin + DMSO (1:1)		720–775 (BF filter)	Kr (674, 676 nm, 5 W) CW rhodamine 6G laser (2.5 W) several 10 mW	0.4 W	18
DMSO	0.008	695 (etalon)	Fl rhodamine B laser (620 nm, 200 ns, 130 mJ) + Ruby (5 J, 25 ns) pumped amplifier	E = 6% 1 J, 45 MW	19

#M11 3,3'-Diethyl-6,6'-dimethoxythiadicarbocyanine iodide; NK 1129

EG	0.1	756 (BB)	Ruby (25 MW, 10–15 ns)	E = 12%	4
DMSO	0.14	710–755 (grating)	Ruby (1.4 MW, 50 ns, 5 Hz)	E = 23%	20

(continued)

31

Table 5 (continued)

Solvent	Concentration (mM)	Lasing wavelength (tuning) (nm)	Excitation	Output	Ref.
#M12 3,3'-Diallyl-5,6,5',6'-tetramethoxythiadicarbocyanine iodide					
Methanol	0.03	~790 (BB)	Ruby (5 MW)		21
#M13 3,3'-Diethyl-5,5'-dimethoxy-6,6'-bis(methylmercapto)-10-methylthiadicarbocyanine bromide					
Ethanol		727–739 (BB, concentration)	Ruby (10 MW/cm^2)		22
#M14 3,3'-Diethyl-10-chloro-4,5,4',5'-dibenzothiadicarbocyanine iodide (p-toluenesulfonate); DC45DTDC; NK 378; NK 460					
Acetone	0.01–0.2	710–720 and 770–779 (BB, concentration)	Ruby (20 MW, 18 ns)	1.5 MW	3
DMSO	200	785 (grating)	N_2 (100 kW, 10 ns, 100 Hz)		16
Methanol	0.1	774 (BB) p-toluenesulf-onate	Ruby (25 MW, 10–15 ns)		4

#M15 3,3'-Diethyl-10-chloro-6,7,6',7'-dibenzothiadicarbocyanine iodide; DC67DTDC; NK 463

Solvent	Conc.	Wavelength	Pump		Ref.
Acetone	0.1	714 (BB)	Ruby (20 MW, 18 ns)		3
Acetone	0.01–0.5	710–716 and 767–772 (BB, concentration)	Ruby (25 MW, 10–15 ns)	E = 11.7%	4
DMSO	100	779 (grating)	N_2 (100 kW, 10 ns, 100 Hz)		16

#M16 3,3'-Diethyl-10-chloro-5,6,5',6'-dibenzothiadicarbocyanine iodide

Solvent	Conc.	Wavelength	Pump		Ref.
Acetone	0.25	720 (BB)	N_2 (400 kW, 10 ns)		23

#M17 3,3'-Diethyloxadicarbocyanine iodide; DODC; DEODC; NK 1533

Solvent	Conc.	Wavelength	Pump		Ref.
Methanol	1	658 (BB)	Glass-SH		24
DMSO	0.2	662 (BB)	Fl (9 J, 80 ns, RT)	Thr = 2.9 J	1
+ Rhodamine B		610–679.5 (grating, concentration)	N_2 (250 kW)	>10 kW	14
Methanol or EG			Mode-locked HeNe (intracavity pump)		12

(continued)

Table 5 *(continued)*

Solvent	Concentration (mM)	Lasing wavelength (tuning) (nm)	Excitation	Output	Ref.
Ethanol + water	1	610–620 (−130 to 15°C) 638–651 (−40 to 20°C)	Glass–SH		25
DMSO	0.2	665 (BB)	Fl (100 J, 100 ns, RT)	Thr = 9 J	11
#M18 1,3,3,1',3',3'-Hexamethylindodicarbocyanine iodide; HIDC; NK 529; hexacyanine					
DMSO	0.2	740 (BB)	Fl (9 J, 80 ns, RT)	Thr = 1.9 J	1
DMSO	0.33	725 (prism)	Fl rhodamine B laser (620 nm, 200 ns, 130 mJ)	E = 3% (75 ns)	19
DMSO	0.2	740	Fl (40 J, 1 μs)		26
#M19 1,3,3,1',3',3'-Hexamethyl-4,5,4',5'-dibenzoindodicarbocyanine iodide					
Ethanol	1	(DFB)	Mode-locked ruby (15–25 mJ, 50–300 ps)		64

34

#M20 1,1'-Diethyl-2,2'-quinodicarbocyanine iodide; DDI; NK 1456

Solvent	Conc.	Wavelength	Pump	Efficiency	Ref.
Glycerin		761–782 (BB, cell length)	Ruby (100 MW)		5
Glycerin	0.063	762 and 806 (BB)	Ruby (100 MW/cm^2)	E = 13%	7
EG	0.1	812 (BB)	Ruby (25 MW, 10–15 ns)	E = 7.8%	4
Glycerin	0.2	740–770 (grating)	Fl (100 J, 100 ns, RT)	Thr = 60 J	11
EG	0.1		Ruby (1.4 MW, 50 ns, 5 Hz)	E = 4%	20
DMSO	0.125–0.25	742–1050 (DFB)	Ruby (130 mJ, 25 ns)	20 mJ, 1.33 MW	27

#M21 1,1'-Dimethyl-11-bromo-2,2'-quinodicarbocyanine iodide; NK 105

Solvent	Conc.	Wavelength	Pump	Efficiency	Ref.
Glycerin	0.1	745 (BB)	Ruby (20 MW, 18 ns)		3

#M22 1,1'-Diethyl-11-bromo-2,2'-quinodicarbocyanine iodide; NK 103

Solvent	Conc.	Wavelength	Pump	Efficiency	Ref.
Glycerin	0.006–0.15	753–775 and 803–819 (BB, concentration)	Ruby (20 MW, 18 ns)	2.7 MW	3

#M23 1,1'-Diethyl-γ-acetoxy-2,2'-dicarbocyanine tetrafluoroborate

Solvent	Conc.	Wavelength	Pump	Efficiency	Ref.
Methanol	0.1	797 (BB)	Ruby (5 MW, 10 ns)		9

(continued)

Table 5 (continued)

Solvent	Concentration (mM)	Lasing wavelength (tuning) (nm)	Excitation	Output	Ref.
#M24 1,1'-Diethyl-γ-cyano-2,2'-dicarbocyanine tetrafluoroborate; DTCDCT					
Methanol	0.1	740 (BB)	Ruby (5 MW, 10 ns)		9
Pyridine	0.1	760–770 (grating)	Ruby (20 MW)	2 MW, E = 10%	28
#M25 1,1'-Diethyl-4,4'-quinodicarbocyanine iodide; NK 1144					
DMSO	0.04–0.8	880–889 and 918–939 (BB, concentration)	Ruby (25 MW, 10–15 ns)	E = 4.9%	4
EG	0.1	930 (BB)	Ruby (25 MW, 10–15 ns)	E = 5.6%	
Methyl sulfoxide	1	930 (BB)	N$_2$ (400 kW, 10 ns)		23
DMSO	0.53	845–920 (grating)	Ruby (1.4 MW, 50 ns, 5 Hz)	E = 25%	20

#M26	1,1'-Diethyl-11-bromo-4,4'-quinodicarbocyanine iodide; NK 104				
Methanol	0.1	830 (BB)	Ruby (20 MW, 18 ns)		3
#M27	1,1'-Diethyl-11-chloro-4,4'-quinodicarbocyanine iodide; NK 78				
EG	0.1	(BB)	Ruby (25 MW, 10-15 ns)	E = 6.0%	4
#M28	1,1'-Diethyl-γ-nitro-4,4'-quinodicarbocyanine tetrafluoroborate; DTNDCT				
Methanol	0.1	796 (BB)	Ruby (5 MW, 10 ns)		9
Ethanol		805 (BB)			
Acetone		814 (BB)			
DMF		815 (BB)			
Pyridine	0.1	~800 (grating)	Ruby (26 MW, 30 ns)	3 MW	28
		812 (BB)	Mode-locked ruby (>150 MW) (synchronous pump)	5 MW	

(continued)

Table 5 (continued)

^aStructures:

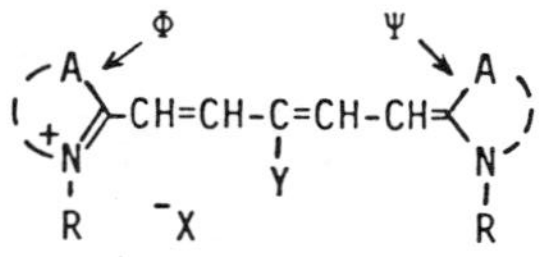

#M10- #M28

Dye no.	Φ; Ψ	R	X	Y	Dye no.	Φ; Ψ	R	X	Y
#M10	(a)	Et	I,ClO$_4$	H	#M20	(s)	Et	I	H
#M11	(b)	Et	I	H	#M21	(s)	Me	I	Br
#M12	(d)	C$_3$H$_5$	I	H	#M22	(s)	Et	I	Br
#M13	(e)	Et	Br	SMe	#M23	(s)	Et	BF$_4$	OAc
#M14	(g)	Et	I,Ts	Cl	#M24	(s)	Et	BF$_4$	CN
#M15	(f)	Et	I	Cl	#M25	(t)	Et	I	H
#M16	(h)	Et	I	Cl	#M26	(t)	Et	I	Br
#M17	(n)	Et	I	H	#M27	(t)	Et	I	Cl
#M18	(p)	Me	I	H	#M28	(t)	Et	BF$_4$	NO$_2$
#M19	(r)	Me	I	H					

Table 6. Tricarbocyanine Dyes and Their Laser Characteristics[a]

Solvent	Concentration (mM)	Lasing wavelength (tuning) (nm)	Excitation	Output	Ref.
#M29 3,3'-Diethylthiatricarbocyanine iodide (bromide); DTTC; NK 126; NK 1666					
Methanol	0.005-1	803-865 (BB, concentration) bromide	Ruby (5 MW, 10 ns)	400 kW	6
Methanol		816 (BB)	Ruby (4.45 MW)	0.63 MW, E = 14%	29
Methanol	0.004-1	793.5-846.5 (BB, concentration)	Ruby (25 MW)	E = 9%	30
DMSO		816 (BB)	Ruby (25 MW)	6.1 MW, E = 25%	
Acetone	0.003-0.4	795-845 (BB, concentration)	Ruby (20 MW, 18 ns)	4 MW	3
DMSO	0.05	881 (BB)	Fl (60 J, 150 ns, RT)	Thr = 48 J (80 ns)	10

(continued)

Table 6 (continued)

Solvent	Concentration (mM)	Lasing wavelength (tuning) (nm)	Excitation	Output	Ref.
DMSO	0.2	889 and 863 (BB)	Fl (9 J, 80 ns, RT)	Thr = 4.6 J	1
DMSO	0.06	790–870.5 (grating + prism)	Ruby (2 MW)	400 kW	31
DMSO	0.1	872 (BB)	Fl (128 J, 700 ns, RT)	3.6 mJ, 9.4 kW	32
DMSO	200	876 (grating)	N_2 (100 kW, 10 ns, 100 Hz)		16
Acetone	0.5	817–840 (grating)	N_2 (300 kW, 10 ns)	0.8–1 ns	17
Glycerin + DMSO (1:1)		840–870 (BF filter)	Kr (674 and 676 nm, 5 W)	60 mW	18
DMSO	0.2	834 (prism)	Carbazine-122 dye laser (700 nm, 8.5 MW, 10 ns, 10 Hz)	220 mWav.	33

		820–900 (grating)	Fl Kiton Red laser (620 nm, 250 ns, 5 kW)	34
EG	1	870–900	Kr (676 and 752.5 nm)	26
DMSO	0.2	860–885	Fl (40 J, 1 μs)	
DMSO	2	865–885 (grating)	N_2 (2 MW, 5 ns)	

#M30 3,3'-Diethyl-11-methoxythiatricarbocyanine iodide

Ethanol		773–798 (BB, concentration)	Ruby (10 MW/cm^2)	22

#M31 3,3'-Diphenylthiatricarbocyanine iodide; IR-116

DMSO	0.1	885 (BB)	Fl (128 J, 700 ns, RT) 2.0 mJ, 6.5 kW	32

#M32 3,3'-Diethyl-5,5'-dimethoxythiatricarbocyanine iodide; NK 1558

EG	0.1	869 (BB)	Ruby (25 MW, 10–15 ns) E = 17.1%	4
DMSO	0.006–0.7	838–893 and 914 (BB, concentration)		

(continued)

Table 6 *(continued)*

Solvent	Concentration (mM)	Lasing wavelength (tuning) (nm)	Excitation	Output	Ref.
DMSO + Acetone	0.1-0.5	820-910 (DFB)	Ruby (12 MW)	1.5 MW	47
DMSO	0.17	820-875 (grating)	Ruby (1.4 MW, 50 ns, 5 Hz)	E = 24%	20

#M33 3,3'-Diethyl-6,6'-dimethoxythiatricarbocyanine iodide; NK 1557

| EG | 0.1 | 878 (BB) | Ruby (25 MW, 10-15 ns) | E = 15% | 4 |

#M34 3,3'-Diethyl-5,6,5',6'-tetramethoxythiatricarbocyanine iodide; NK 428

| Acetone | 0.02-0.4 | 842-887 (BB, concentration) | Ruby (20 MW, 18 ns) | 2 MW | 3 |
| DMSO | 0.3 | 855-885 (grating) | Ruby (1.4 MW, 50 ns, 5 Hz) | E= 19% | 20 |

#M35 3,3'-Diethyl-4,5,4',5'-dibenzothiatricarbocyanine iodide; DDTTC; NK 427; dibenzocyanine 45

| Acetone | 0.003-0.4 | 838-886 (BB, concentration) | Ruby (20 MW, 18 ns) | 2.1 MW | 3 |

Solvent	Concentration	Wavelength (nm)	Pump laser	Output	Ref.
DMSO	0.01–0.5	866–886 and 914–928 (BB, concentration)	Ruby (25 MW, 10–15 ns)	E = 8.8%	4
DMSO	0.06	834–900 (grating + prism)	Ruby (2 MW)	350 kW	31
DMSO	200	928 (grating)	N_2 (100 kW, 10 ns, 100 Hz)		16
Acetone	0.5	870 (BB)	N_2 (400 kW, 10 ns)		23
DMSO	2	905–940 (grating)	N_2 (2 MW, 5 ns)		26
DMSO + DTTC (3:50)	2.5	875–905 (grating)			
DMSO	1.5	899–975 (grating)	Excimer (XeCl)	E = 3%	

#M36 3,3'-Diethyl-6,7,6',7'-dibenzothiatricarbocyanine iodide; NK 1887

Solvent	Concentration	Wavelength (nm)	Pump laser	Output	Ref.
Ethanol		824–853 (BB, concentration)	Ruby (10 MW/cm^2)		22

(continued)

Table 6 (continued)

Solvent	Concentration (mM)	Lasing wavelength (tuning) (nm)	Excitation	Output	Ref.
#M37 3,3'-Diethyl-6,7,6',7'-dibenzo-11-methylthiatricarbocyanine iodide					
Ethanol		843–869 (BB, concentration)	Ruby (10 MW/cm^2)		22
#M38 3,3'-Diethyl-5,5'-dimethylthiazolinotricarbocyanine iodide					
DMSO	200	745 (grating)	N$_2$ (100 kW, 10 ns, 100 Hz)		16
#M39 3,5,3',5'-Tetramethylthiazolinotricarbocyanine iodide; NK 746					
Glycerin	0.1	717 (BB)	Ruby (20 MW, 18 ns)		3
EG	0.1	725 (BB)	Ruby (25 MW, 10–15 ns)	E = 13.1%	4
#M40 3-Ethyl-3'-methylthiathiazolinotricarbocyanine iodide; NK 1818					
Ethanol		738–801 (BB, concentration)	Ruby (10 MW/cm^2)		22

#M41 3,5,3',5'-Tetramethylthiathiazolinotricarbocyanine iodide

DMSO	0.41	710–765 (grating)	Ruby (1.4 MW, 50 ns, 5 Hz)	E = 43%	20

#M42 3,3'-Diethylselenatricarbocyanine iodide; DSTC; NK 747

Acetone	0.1	826 (BB)	Ruby (20 MW, 18 ns)		3
Methanol	0.025	825 (BB)	Ruby (5 MW)		21
EG	0.1	850 (BB)	Ruby (25 MW, 10–15 ns)	E = 2.9%	4
DMSO + rhodamine B (2:50)	2	865 (grating)	N_2 (100 kW, 10 ns, 100 Hz)		16

#M43 3,3'-Dimethyloxatricarbocyanine iodide DOTC; DMOTC; methyl DOTC; NK 199

Acetone	0.004–0.4	720–770 (BB, concentration)	Ruby (20 MW, 18 ns)	4 MW	3
DMSO	0.2	809 (BB)	Fl (9 J, 80 ns, RT)	Thr = 1.9 J	1
Water + Triton X-100 (1.5%)	0.2	740–787 (grating)	Ruby (20 MW, 40 ns)		15
DMSO	0.2	780–820 (grating)	Fl (100 J, 100 ns, RT)	Thr = 7.3 J, E = 0.06%	11

(continued)

45

Table 6 (continued)

Solvent	Concentration (mM)	Lasing wavelength (tuning) (nm)	Excitation	Output	Ref.
DMSO (SA:HITC)		795–805 (grating)	Fl (100 J, 100 ns, RT) mode locking		11
DMSO	100	782 (BB)	N_2 (100 kW, 10 ns, 100 Hz)		16
EG	~3	745–790 (BF filter)	Kr (647.1 nm, 0.75 W)		35
DMSO	0.2	749 (BB)	Carbazine-122 dye laser (700 nm, 10.5 MW, 10 Hz)	470 mWav. E = 45%	36
DMSO	0.05–0.1	769 (etalon)	Ruby (2.8 J, 15 ns) (osc + amp)	1 J, E = 47%	37
DMSO deoxygenated + N-aminohomo-piperidine (0.6%)	0.15	810 (IF filter)	Fl (150 J + 720 J) (osc + amp)	0.1 J, 1 μs	38

Solvent	Concentration	Tuning range (nm)	Pump source	Output	Ref.
DMSO + EG (1:3)	1	745–860 (BF filter)	Kr (647 nm, 1.1 W, 200 ps) (synchronous pumping)	90 mW (3–70 ps)	39
Glycerin + DMSO (1:1) + COT		752–864 (BF filter)	Kr (647 and 676 nm, 5 W)	1 W	18
DMSO	1	765–795 (grating)	N_2 (2 MW, 5 ns)		26
DMSO	4.8	779–830 (grating)	Excimer (XeCl)	E = 2%	

#M44 3,3'-Diethyloxatricarbocyanine iodide; DOTC; DEOTC; NK 1511

Solvent	Concentration	Tuning range (nm)	Pump source	Output	Ref.
Ethanol	0.1	718–739 (BB, concentration)	Ruby (10 MW/cm^2)		22
Acetone	0.002–0.07	742 (BB)	Ruby (20 MW, 18 ns)		3
Methanol		722–770 (BB, concentration)	Ruby .(5 MW)	0.73 MW	21
DMSO	250	788.4 (grating)	N_2 (100 kW, 10 ns, 100 Hz)		16
Acetone	0.5	732–758 (grating)	N_2 (300 kW, 10 ns)	0.8–1 ns	17

(continued)

47

Table 6 *(continued)*

Solvent	Concentration (mM)	Lasing wavelength (tuning) (nm)	Excitation	Output	Ref.
	2	765–790 (grating)	N_2 (300 kW, 10 ns)		17
Glycerin + DMSO (1:1) + COT	1	757–872 (BF filter)	Kr (647 and 676 nm, 5 W)	1.6 W	18
Acetone	0.08–0.04	763.9 (grating)	Ruby (5 J, 2.5 GW)	1.1 J, 0.55 GW	40
DMSO	0.1	745 (etalon)	Fl rhodamine B laser (620 nm, 200 ns, 130 mJ)	E = 7%	19
DMSO + EG (1:1)	1	760–870	Kr (647, 676 nm)		26
DMSO	0.2	785–840	Fl (40 J, 1 μs)		
DMSO	2.5	780–800 (grating)	N_2 (2 MW, 5 ns)		
		760–840 (etalon)	Kr (647, 676 nm, 4 W)	0.6 W	41

#M45 3,3'-Diethyl-5,6,5',6'-tetramethyloxatricarbocyanine iodide; NK 1241

#M46 1,3,3,1',3',3'-Hexamethylindotricarbocyanine iodide (perchlorate); HITC; NK 125; hexacyanine 3

EG	0.1	787 (BB)	Ruby (25 MW, 10–15 ns)	E = 11%	4
Ethanol		779–808 (BB, concentration)	Ruby (10 MW/cm^2)		22
Methanol	0.003–0.4	775–842 (BB, concentration)	Ruby (20 MW, 18 ns)	4 MW	3
DMSO	0.06	780–883 (grating + prism)	Ruby (2 MW)	320 kW	31
DMSO	200	861.6 (BB)	N_2 (100 kW, 10 ns, 100 Hz)		16
DMSO	0.5	849 (BB)	YAG-SH (10 ns, 25–40 mJ, 10–30 Hz)	E = 2%	42
EG	0.8 g/l	834–889 (BF filter)	Kr (647 and 676 nm, 1.5 W)	42 mW	43
DMSO	0.2	822 (prism)	Carbazine-122 dye laser (700 nm, 8.5 MW, 10 ns, 10 Hz)	210 mWav.	33

(continued)

Table 6 (continued)

Solvent	Concentration (mM)	Lasing wavelength (tuning) (nm)	Excitation	Output	Ref.
DMSO + EG (1:3)	1	835–905 (BF filter)	Kr (647 nm, 1.1 W, 200 ps) (synchronous pumping)	50 mW (3–70 ps)	39
Glycerin + DMSO (1:4)	1.3	828–909 (BF filter)	Kr (674 and 676 nm, 5 W)	0.4 W	18
Glycerin + DMSO (1:4)	0.4	812–929 (BF filter)	Kr (752 and 799 nm, 2 W)	0.25 W	
DMSO	0.2	879 (BB)	Fl (100 J, 100 ns, RT)	Thr = 9 J	11
DMSO (SA:DTC)		872–880 (grating)	Fl (100 J, 100 ns, RT) mode locking		
DMSO (SA:DTTC)		857–863 (grating)	Fl (100 J, 100 ns, RT) mode locking		
DMSO + EG (1:1)	1	830–940	Kr (647–799 nm)		26
DMSO	2	845–870 (grating)	N_2 (2 MW, 5 ns)		

Solvent	Conc.	Tuning range (nm)	Pump	Output	
DMSO	2.2	837–905 (grating)	Excimer (XeCl)		E = 4%
		820–876 (etalon) perchlorate	Kr (647 and 676 nm, 4 W)	0.5 W	41
EG + DMSO (4:1)		840–895 (single axial mode, ring cavity)	Kr (all red lines, 8.3 W)	140 mW	303

#M47 1,3,3,1',3',3'-Hexamethyl-6,7,6',7'-dibenzoindotricarbocyanine perchlorate; HDITC; hexadibenzocyanine 3

Solvent	Conc.	Tuning range (nm)	Pump	Output	
Glycerin + DMSO (1:4) + COT	0.7	879–964 (BF filter)	Kr (752 and 799 nm, 2 W)	100 mW	18
DMSO + EG (1:1) + COT	0.7	885–960	Kr (676 and 752 nm)		26

#M48 1,3,3,1',3',3'-Hexamethyl-4,5,4',5'-dibenzoindotricarbocyanine perchlorate

Solvent	Conc.	Tuning range (nm)	Pump	Output	
Ethanol		816–833 (BB, concentration)	Ruby (10 MW/cm^2)		22

(continued)

Table 6 (continued)

Solvent	Concentration (mM)	Lasing wavelength (tuning) (nm)	Excitation	Output	Ref.
#M49 3,3,3',3'-Tetramethyl-1,1'-di (4-sulfobutyl)-4,5,4',5'-dibenzo-indotricarbocyanine iodide, monosodium salt; IR-125					
DMSO	0.03-1	924-952 (BB, concentration)	F1 (128 J, 700 ns, RT)	16 mJ, 34 kW	32
DMSO	0.5	913 (BB)	YAG-SH (10 ns, 25-40 mJ, 10-30 Hz)	E = 2.6%	42
DMSO	0.23	840-920 (grating)	Ruby (1.4 MW, 50 ns, 5 Hz)	E = 14%	20
DMSO	0.2	903 (prism)	Carbazine-122 dye laser (700 nm, 8.5 MW, 10 ns, 10 Hz)	180 mWav.	33
#M50 1,1'-Diethyl-2,2'-quinotricarbocyanine iodide; NK 123					
Ethanol		886-898 (BB, concentration)	Ruby (10 MW/cm^2)		22

Acetone	0.025-0.5	880-962 (BB, concentration)	Ruby (20 MW, 18 ns)	1 MW	3
DMSO	0.025-1	915-969 (BB, concentration)	Ruby (25 MW, 10-15 ns)	E = 6.2%	4
DMSO	0.08	865-920 (grating + prism)	Ruby (2 MW)	100 kW	31

#M51 1,1'-Diethyl-4,4'-quinotricarbocyanine iodide; NK 124

Acetone	0.02-1	983-1060 (BB, concentration)	Ruby (20 MW, 18 ns)	1.3 MW	3
DMSO	0.03-1	1020-1083 (BB, concentration)	Ruby (25 MW, 10-15 ns)	E = 6.2%	4
Acetone	1	970-1125 (grating)	Ruby (25 MW, 25 ns)	1.2 MW	44
DMSO	2.5	1020-1145 (grating)	Ruby (25 MW, 25 ns)	2 MW	
DMSO		1030-1096 (BB, concentration)	IR N_2 (0.92-1.09 µm, 0.6 mJ, 150 ns, 40 Hz)	E = 5%	45

(continued)

Table 6 (continued)

Solvent	Concentration (mM)	Lasing wavelength (tuning) (nm)	Excitation	Output	Ref.
#M52 3,3'-Diethyl-9,11-neopentylenethiatricarbocyanine iodide					
DMSO	0.2	880 (BB)	Fl (100 J, 100 ns, RT)	Thr = 11 J	11
#M53 3,3'-Diethyl-10,12-ethylene-11-(N-methylanilinothiatricarbocyanine perchlorate; IR-137					
DMSO	0.1	950 (BB)	Fl (128 J, 700 ns, RT)	30 mJ, 42 kW	32
DMSO + EG (1:2)	0.8 g/l	855–1032 (BF filter)	Kr (752 nm, 0.5 W) (synchronous pumping)	110 mW	46
#M54 3,3'-Diethyl-10,12-ethylene-11-morpholinothiatricarbocyanine iodide; IR-109					
DMSO	0.1	875 (BB)	Fl (128 J, 700 ns, RT)	8.6 mJ, 17 kW	32

#M55 5,5'-Dichloro-3,3'-diethyl-10,12-ethylene-11-(N-methylanilino)-thiatricarbocyanine iodide; IR-141

DMSO	0.1	946 (BB)	Fl (128 J, 700 ns, RT)	3.7 mJ, 12 kW	32

#M56 5,5'-Dichloro-11-diphenylamino-3,3'-diethyl-10,12-ethylene-thiatricarbocyanine perchlorate; IR-140

Tetra-methylene sulfoxide	1-2	950-1005 (BB, concentration)	GaAlAs diode (820 nm, 50 ns, 9 Wav., 200 Hz)	220 mWav.	48
DMSO	0.1	950 (BB)	Fl (128 J, 700 ns, RT)	53 mJ, 63 kW	32
DMSO	0.5	910 (BB)	YAG-SH (10 ns, 25-40 mJ, 10-30 Hz)	E = 9%	42
Methyl sulfoxide	0.2	865-890 (grating)	N_2 (300 kW, 10 ns)	0.8-1 ns	17
	2	900-925 (grating)			
	5	935-960 (grating)			

(continued)

Table 6 (continued)

Solvent	Concentration (mM)	Lasing wavelength (tuning) (nm)	Excitation	Output	Ref.
DMSO	0.2	898 (prism)	Carbazine-122 dye laser (700 nm, 8.5 MW, 10 ns, 10 Hz)	170 mWav.	33
DMSO + EG (1:3)	0.4 g/l	890-985 (BF filter)	Kr (752 and 799 nm, 2.7 W, 200 ps) (synchronous pumping)	250 mW (3-70 ps)	39
DMSO + EG (1:1)	0.5 g/l	862-1013 (BF filter)	Kr (752 and 799 nm, 2 W)	250 mW	49
DMSO + EG (1:2)	0.8 g/l	858-1030 (BF filter)	Kr (752 nm, 0.5 W) (synchronous pumping)	100 mW	46
DMSO		918-968 (BB, concentration) 919-988 (grating)	IR N_2 (0.92-1.09 μm, 0.6 mJ, 150 ns, 40 Hz)	E = 20%	45

#M57 11-Dimethylamino-3,3'-diethyl-10,12-ethylene-4,5,4'',5'-dibenzo-thiatricarbocyanine perchlorate; IR-139

DMSO	0.1	883 (BB)	Fl (128 J, 700 ns, RT)	9.3 mJ, 17 kW	32

#M58 11-Diphenylamino-3,3'-diethyl-10,12-ethylene-4,5,4'',5'-dibenzo-thiatricarbocyanine perchlorate; IR-143

DMSO	0.1	972 (BB)	Fl (128 J, 700 ns, RT)	8.1 mJ, 18 kW	32
DMSO + EG (1:1)	0.8 g/l	913-1020 (BF filter)	Kr (752 and 799 nm, 2 W)	35 mW	49
DMSO + EG (1:2)	0.8 g/l	894-1095 (BF filter)	Kr (752 nm, 0.5 W) (synchronous pumping)	50 mW	46

#M59 11-(4-Ethoxycarbonylpiperidino)-3,3'-diethyl-10,12-ethylene-4,5,4'',5'-dibenzothiatricarbocyanine perchlorate; IR-134

DMSO	0.1	888 (BB)	Fl (128 J, 700 ns, RT)	1.7 mJ, 6.7 kW	32

#M60 3,3'-Di (3-acetoxpropyl)-11-diphenylamino-10,12-ethylene-5,6,5',6'-dibenzothiatricarbocyanine perchlorate; IR-132

DMSO	0.03-0.1	957-972 (BB, concentration)	Fl (128 and 700 ns, RT)	6.4 mJ, 20 kW	32

57

(continued)

Table 6 (continued)

Solvent	Concentration (mM)	Lasing wavelength (tuning) (nm)	Excitation	Output	Ref.
DMSO	0.5	909.5 (BB)	YAG-SH (10 ns, 25–40 mJ, 10–30 Hz)	E = 1.3%	42
DMSO	0.12	875–920 (grating)	Ruby (1.4 MW, 50 ns, 5 Hz)	E = 7%	20
DMSO + EG (1:3)	0.4 g/l	910–980 (BF filter)	Kr (752 and 799 nm, 2.7 W, 200 ps) (synchronous pumping)	50 mW (3–70 ps)	39
DMSO + EG (1:2)	0.8 g/l	863–1048 (BF filter)	Kr (752 nm, 0.5 W) (synchronous pumping)	Thr = 30 mW	46

#M61 3'-Ethyl-10,12-ethylene-1,3,3-trimethyl-11-(1-pyrrolidinyl)-indothiatricarbocyanine iodide; IR-136

Solvent	Concentration (mM)	Lasing wavelength (tuning) (nm)	Excitation	Output	Ref.
DMSO	0.1		Fl (128 J, 700 ns, RT)	1.5 mJ, 6 kW	32

#M62 11-(4-Ethoxycarbonyl-1-piperazinyl)-3,3'-diethyl-10,12-ethylene-5,5'-diphenyl-oxatricarbocyanine perchlorate; IR-145

DMSO	0.1		Fl (128 J, 700 ns, RT)	4 mJ, 7.3 kW	32

#M63 Anhydro-11-(4-ethoxycarbonyl-1-piperazinyl)-10,12-ethylene-3,3,3',3'-tetramethyl-1,1'-di(3-sulfopropyl)-4,5,4',5'-dibenzo-indotricarbocyanine hydroxide, triethylammonium salt; IR-144

DMSO	0.1	880 and 945 (BB)	Fl (128 J, 700 ns, RT)	22-33 mJ, 28-42 kW	32
DMSO	0.5	869 (BB)	YAG-SH (10 ns, 25-40 mJ, 10-30 Hz)	E = 11%	42
DMSO	0.22	835-890 (grating)	Ruby (1.4 MW, 50 ns, 5 Hz)	E = 21%	20
DMSO	0.2	844-885 (prism)	Carbazine-122 dye laser (700 nm, 8.5 MW, 10 ns, 10 Hz)	340 mWav. E = 40%	33
DMSO + EG (1:3)	0.4 g/l	840-890 (BF filter)	Kr (752 and 799 nm, 2.7 W, 200 ps) (synchronous pumping)	200 mW (3-70 ps)	39

(continued)

Table 6 *(continued)*

Solvent	Concentration (mM)	Lasing wavelength (tuning) (nm)	Excitation	Output	Ref.
DMSO + EG (1:3)	0.4 g/l	850–980	Cu (510.5 and 578.2 nm, 100 kW, 25 ns, 6 kHz)	E = 7%	50

#M64 2-[3-(3-Ethyl-2-benzothiazolinylidene)methyl]-4-[3-(3-ethyl-2-benzothiazolinylidene) propenyl]-5,6-benzopyrylium iodide; IR-123

Solvent	Concentration (mM)	Lasing wavelength (tuning) (nm)	Excitation	Output	Ref.
DMSO	0.1	835 (BB)	Fl (128 J, 700 ns, RT)	4.4 mJ, 13.3 kW	32
DMSO	0.16	765–815 (grating)	Ruby (1.4 MW, 50 ns, 5 Hz)	E = 22%	20
DMSO	0.2	768–819 (prism)	Carbazine-122 dye laser (700 nm, 8.5 MW, 10 ns, 10 Hz)	280 mWav.	33

#M65 4-[3-(3-Ethyl-2-benzothiazolinylidene) propenyl]-2-[(3-ethyl-2-benzoxazolinylidene) methyl]-5,6-benzopyrylium iodide; IR-135

DMSO	0.1	810 (BB)	F1 (128 J, 700 ns, RT)	2.1 mJ, 6.5 kW	32

^{a} Structures (see also Table 9):

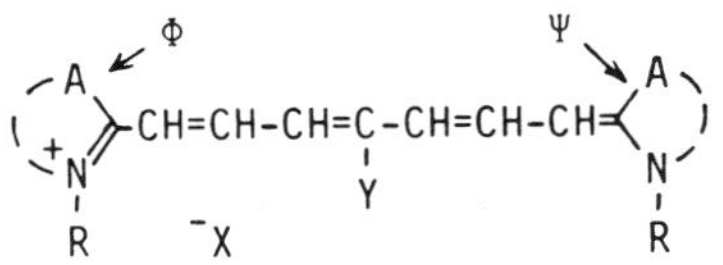

#M52

#M29 — #M51

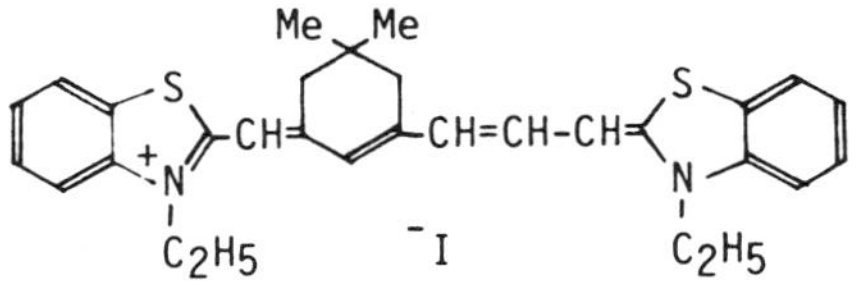

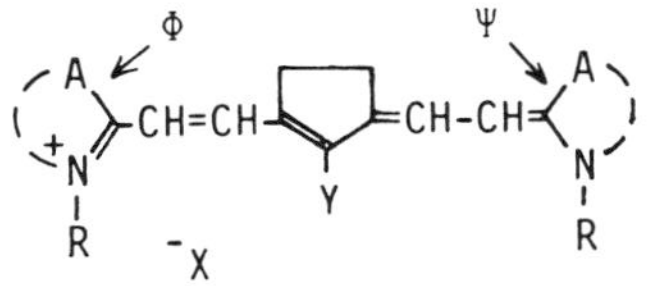

#M53 — #M63

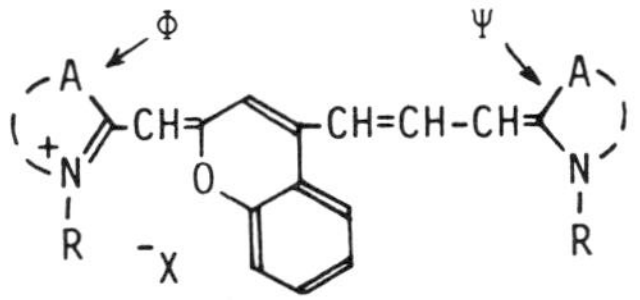

#M64, 65

(continued)

61

Table 6 (continued)

Dye no.	Φ; Ψ	R	X	Y
#M29	(a)	Et	I,Br	H
#M30	(a)	Et	I	OMe
#M31	(a)	Ph	I	H
#M32	(c)	Et	I	H
#M33	(b)	Et	I	H
#M34	(d)	Et	I	H
#M35	(g)	Et	I	H
#M36	(f)	Et	I	H
#M37	(f)	Et	I	Me
#M38	(m)	Et	I	H
#M39	(m)	Me	I	H
#M40	(a); (l)	Et;Me	I	H
#M41	(k); (m)	Me	I	H
#M42	(u)	Et	I	H

Dye no.	Φ; Ψ	R	X	Y
#M50	(s)	Et	I	H
#M51	(t)	Et	I	H
#M52		See figure		
#M53	(a)	Et	ClO_4	NMePh
#M54	(a)	Et	I	N⟨⟩O
#M55	(i)	Et	I	NMePh
#M56	(i)	Et	ClO_4	NPh_2
#M57	(g)	Et	ClO_4	NMe_2
#M58	(g)	Et	ClO_4	NPh_2
#M59	(g)	Et	ClO_4	N⟨⟩CO_2Et
#M60	(h)	$(CH_2)_3$OAc	ClO_4	NPh_2
#M61	(a); (p)	Et;Me	I	N⟨⟩

#M43	(n)	Me	I	H
#M44	(n)	Et	I	H
#M45	(o)	Et	I	H
#M46	(p)	Me	I, ClO_4	H
#M47	(q)	Me	ClO_4	H
#M48	(r)	Me	ClO_4	H
#M49	(r)	$(CH_2)_4SO_3^-$ (mono-sodium salt)	I	H

#M62	(j)	Et	ClO_4	N‒CO_2Et
#M63	(r)	$(CH_2)_3SO_3^-$ (HNEt$_3$ salt)	I	N‒CO_2Et
#M64	(a)	Et	I	—
#M65	(a);(n)	Et	I	—

Table 7. Tetracarbocyanine Dyes and Their Laser Characteristics[a]

Solvent	Concentration (mM)	Lasing wavelength (tuning) (nm)	Excitation	Output	Ref.
#M66 3,3'-Diethyl-12-acetoxythiatetracarbocyanine perchlorate; DaTTeC; NK 1748					
DMSO	0.01–1	948–1018 (BB, concentration)	Ruby (25 MW, 10–15 ns)	E = 14.6%	4
DMSO	0.08	920–950 (grating)	Ruby (1.4 MW, 50 ns, 5 Hz)	E = 20%	20
		945–1023 (BB)	IR N_2 (0.92–1.09 µm,	E = 10%	45
		936–1041 (grating)	0.6 mJ, 150 ns, 40 Hz)		
DMSO + EG (1:1) deoxygenized	0.5 g/l	935–1019 (BF filter)	Kr (752 and 799 nm, 2 W)	30 mW	49
DMSO + EG (1:2)	0.8 g/l	915–1058 (BF filter)	Kr (752 nm, 0.5 W) (synchronous pumping)	30 mW	46

#M67 3,3'-Diethyl-12-ethylthiatetracarbocyanine iodide

| Ethanol | 916–924 (BB, concentration) | Ruby (10 MW/cm^2) | 22 |

#M68 1,1'-Diethyl-13-acetoxy-2,2'-quinotetracarbocyanine perchlorate; NK 1161

| DMSO | 0.05–1 | 1031–1096 (BB, concentration) | Ruby (25 MW, 10–15 ns) | E = 3.3% | 4 |
| DMSO | 1.4 | 1.6 MW | 1020–1140 (grating) | Ruby (25 MW, 25 ns) | 44 |

[a] Structures (see also Table 9):

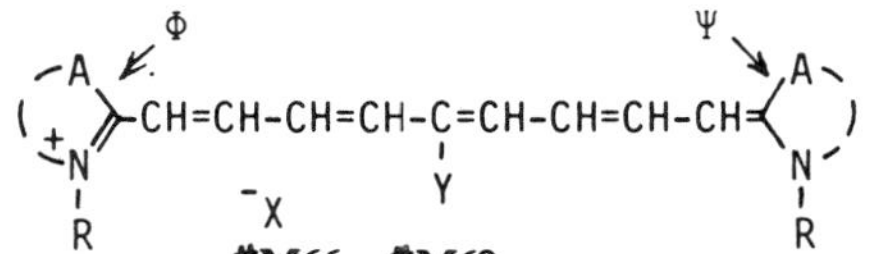

#M66— #M68

Dye no.	Φ; Ψ	R	X	Y
#M66	(a)	Et	ClO$_4$	OAc
#M67	(a)	Et	I	Et
#M68	(s)	Et	ClO$_4$	OAc

Table 8. Pentacarbocyanine Dyes and Their Laser Characteristics[a]

#M69 3,3'-Diethyl-9,11,15,17-dineopentylenethiapentacarbocyanine iodide (perchlorate); DNTPC; NK 2184; NK 2545; DNP-1020

Solvent	Concentration (mM)	Lasing wavelength (tuning) (nm)	Excitation	Output	Ref.
Nitrobenzene		1092.5 (BB)	Glass (50 MW/cm^2)		51
Methanol		1100 (BB)	Ruby		52
DMSO	0.1	1102-1148 (prism)	YAG (20 MW, 12 ns, 10 Hz)	390 mWav.	53
DMSO	1.5 g/l	1100 (grating)	YAG (40 mJ, 18 ns, 10 Hz)	E = 20%	54

#M70 3,3'-Diethyl-9,11,15,17-dineopentylene-5,6,5',6'-tetramethoxy-thiapentacarbocyanine perchlorate; DNXTPC; DNP-1030

Solvent	Concentration (mM)	Lasing wavelength (tuning) (nm)	Excitation	Output	Ref.
DMSO	0.1	1107-1187 (prism)	YAG (50 MW, 12 ns)	3.5 MW, 340 mWav.	55
DMSO	2	1192-1285 (prism)	YAG (50 MW, 12 ns)	1 MW, 90 mWav.	

#M71 3,3'-Diethyl-9,11,15,17-dineopentylene-6,7,6',7'-dibenzo-
thiapentacarbocyanine perchlorate; DNDTPC; DNP-1040

DMSO	0.1	1151–1198 (prism)	YAG (20 MW, 12 ns, 10 Hz)	320 mWav.	53
DMSO	0.15	1084–1125 (prism)	YAG (0.7 J, 15 ns, 8 Hz) (osc + amp)	13 MW, 1 mWav. E = 30%	56
DMSO	0.15	1080–1120 (prism)	YAG (40 mJ, 25 ps, 9–10 pulses) (synchronous pumping)	4 mJ <10 ps, 4–5 pulses	57
DMSO	1.5 g/1	1080–1200 (grating)	YAG (40 mJ, 18 ns, 10 Hz)	0.25 mJ	54
DMSO	0.3	1090–1120 (grating) (osc + amp)	YAG (400 mJ, 10 ns)	20 mJ	310

#M72 3,3'-Diethyl-9,11,15,17-dineopentylene-5,6,5',6'-tetramethyl-
selenapentacarbocyanine perchlorate; DNSPC

DMSO	0.1	1076–1147 (prism)	YAG (50 MW, 12 ns, 10 Hz)	2.9 MW, 290 mW	55

(continued)

Table 8 (continued)

Solvent	Concentration (mM)	Lasing wavelength (tuning) (nm)	Excitation	Output	Ref.
		#M73 Pentacarbocyanine derivative			
Nitrobenzene	$10^{16}-10^{17}$ cm^{-3}	1095-1115 and 1155-1175 (BB, concentration)	Glass (18 MW/cm^2, 25 ns)	0.25 J E = 25%	58

[a] Structures

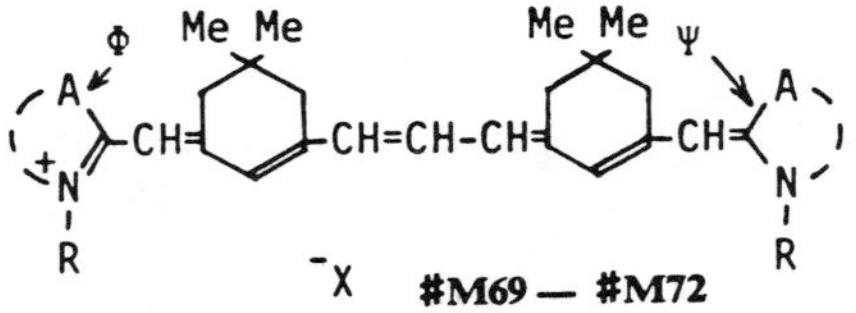

Dye no.	Φ; Ψ		R	X
#M69	(a)		Et	I,ClO$_4$
#M70	(d)		Et	ClO$_4$
#M71	(f)		Et	ClO$_4$
#M72	(v)		Et	ClO$_4$

68

Table 9. Abbreviations Used in Tables 4-8[a]

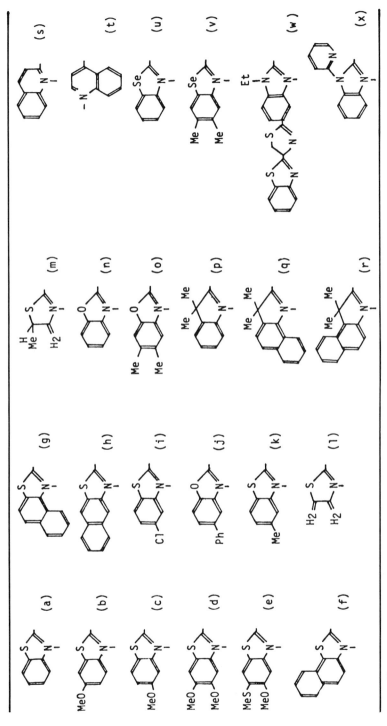

[a]See also Refs. 300, 301 about new cyanine dyes.

Table. 10. Laser Characteristics of Merocyanine Dyes[a]

Solvent	Concentration (mM)	Lasing wavelength (tuning) (nm)	Excitation	Output	Ref.
#M74 3-Ethyl-5-[6-(3-ethyl-2-benzothiazolylidene)-2,4-hexadienylidene]rhodanine; NK 1575					
DMSO	0.1	788 (BB)	Ruby (25 MW, 10-15 ns)		4
#M75 Methyl-1-[6-(3-ethyl-2-benzothiazolylidene)-2,4-hexadienylidene]cyanoacetate; NK 1583					
DMSO	0.1	725 (BB)	Ruby (25 MW, 10-15 ns)		4
#M76 6-(3-Ethyl-2-benzothiazolylidene)-2,4-hexadienylidene thioindogenid; merocyanine B; NK 1586					
DMSO	0.01-1	798-847 (BB, concentration)	Ruby (25 MW, 10-15 ns)	E = 10.9%	4
DMSO	0.13	780-823 (grating)	Ruby (1.4 MW, 50 ns, 5 Hz)	E = 5%	20

#M77 4-{2,5-Di[(3-ethyl-2-benzothiazolinylidene) ethylidene]cyclopentylidene}-1,2-diphenyl-3,5-pyrazolidinedione; IR-107

Solvent	Conc	Tuning (nm)	Pump	Output	Ref
DMSO	0.1	940 (BB)	Fl (128 J, 700 ns, RT)	0.9 mJ, 5 kW	32

#M78 4-Dicyanomethylene-2-methyl-6-p-dimethylaminostyryl-4H-pyran; DCM

Solvent	Conc	Tuning (nm)	Pump	Output	Ref
DMSO	2.6	625–688 (grating) (osc + amp)	Cu (510.6 nm, 2.15 Wav., 32 ns, 6 kHz)	0.43 Wav., E = 18.7%	66
DMSO		610–710 (grating)	N_2 (2 mJ, 8 ns, 5 Hz)	75 µJ	67
DMF		649 (BB)	Fl (5 J)	4.4 mJ	
DMSO		655 (BB)	Fl (5 J)	4.6 mJ	
DMSO	2	632–690 (grating) (osc + amp)	XeCl (150 mJ, 10–20 ns)	E = 10%	26
DMSO	2	615–705 (grating)	N_2 (1.5 MW, 4 ns)		

(continued)

Table 10 *(continued)*

Solvent	Concentration (mM)	Lasing wavelength (tuning) (nm)	Excitation	Output	Ref.
EG + ammonyx LO + benzyl alcohol + COT		610–710 (single axial mode ring cavity)	Ar (all lines, 20 W) Ar (488 nm, 6 W)	2.9 W 0.82 W	303
Benzyl alcohol + EG (4:6)	1.5	605–725 (etalon)	Ar (488 nm, 2 W) mode-locked Ar (514 nm)	690 mW, E = 34% 520 W$_{peak}$ (1.5 ps) (synchronous pumping)	297

[a] Structures:

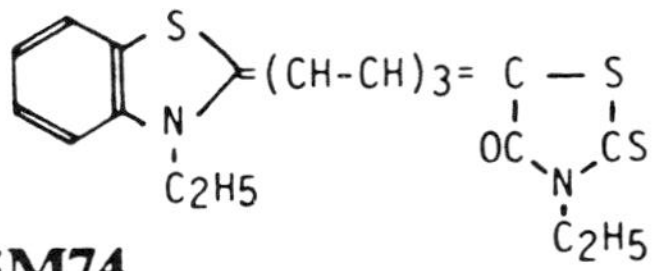

#M74

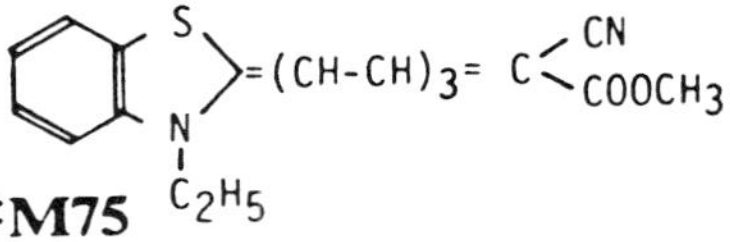

$S \diagup (CH-CH)_3 = C - S$
$OC-N \diagdown^{CS}_{C_2H_5}$
$N-C_2H_5$

#M75

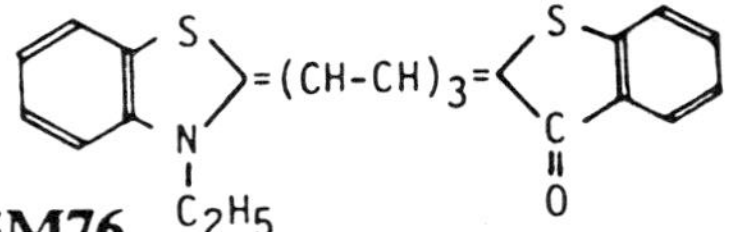

$S \diagup (CH-CH)_3 = C \diagup^{CN}_{COOCH_3}$
$N-C_2H_5$

#M76

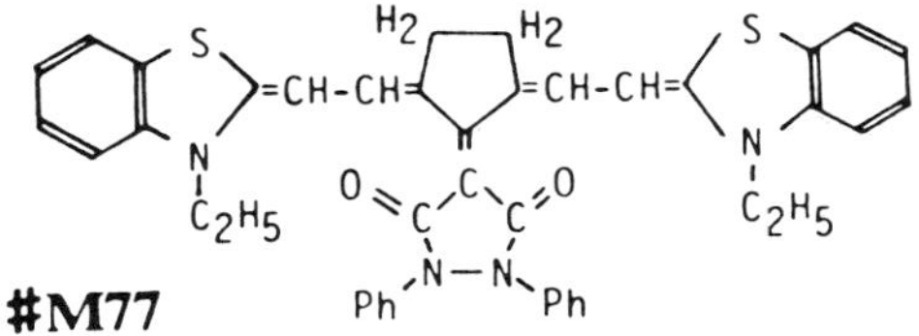

$S \diagup (CH-CH)_3 = C=O$
$N-C_2H_5$

#M77

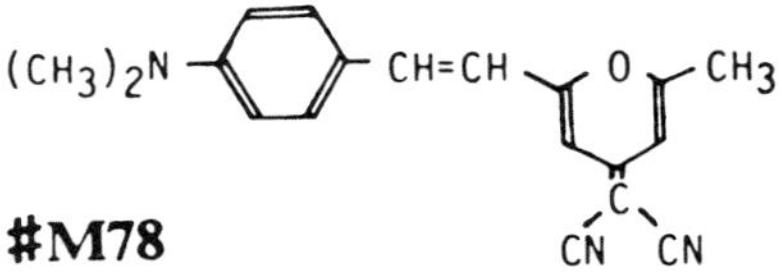

$S \diagup =CH-CH \diagdown$
$N-C_2H_5$
H_2 H_2
$=CH-CH$
$O=C-C \diagup^{C=O}_{N-N-Ph}$
$Ph-N-N$

#M78

$(CH_3)_2N$ —CH=CH— O —CH$_3$
$C \diagdown^{CN}_{CN}$

73

Table 11. Laser Characteristics of Phthalocyanine Dyes[a]

Solvent	Concentration (mM)	Lasing wavelength (tuning) (nm)	Excitation	Ref.
#M79 Metal-free phthalocyanine				
Sulfric acid	5×10^{16}–10^{17} cm^{-3}	863.4 and 755.5 (BB)	Ruby (0.5 J, 30–40 ns)	6
#M80 Magnesium phthalocyanine				
Quinoline	5×10^{16}–10^{17} cm^{-3}	759 (BB)	Ruby (0.5 J, 30–40 ns)	6
Pyridine	1.2	688.2 (BB)	N$_2$ (1 MW, 8 ns)	68
DMF	0.5	682.5 (BB)	N$_2$ (1 MW, 8 ns)	
#M81 Zinc phthalocyanine				
Pyridine	0.5	686 (BB)	N$_2$ (1 MW, 8 ns)	68
#M82 Chloroaluminum phthalocyanine				
Ethanol	5×10^{16}–2×10^{17} cm^{-3}	755 (BB)	Ruby (100 MW/cm^2)	69

1-Propanol	~1	755 (BB)	Ruby (10 MW)	30
DMSO	~1	761.5 (BB)	Ruby (10 MW)	
EG	~1	763 (BB)	Ruby (10 MW)	
Chloronaphthalene	0.06	708 (BB)	Ruby (10 MW, 20 ns)	175
Methanol	1	690 (BB)	N_2 (400 kW, 10 ns)	23
Ethanol	1	753.3 and 685.7 (BB)	N_2 (1 MW, 8 ns)	68
Pyridine	0.28	694 (BB)	N_2 (1 MW, 8 ns)	68

#M83 Gallium pathalocyanine chloride

a Structures:

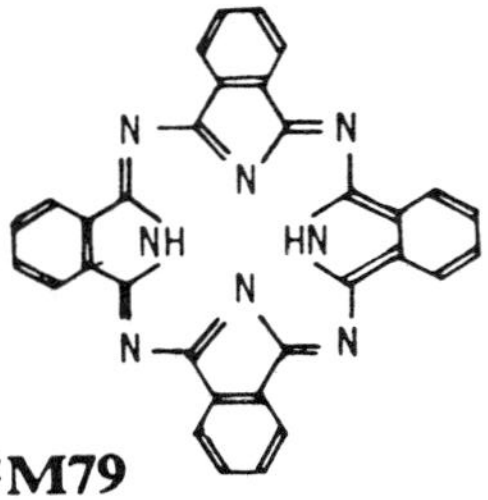

#M79

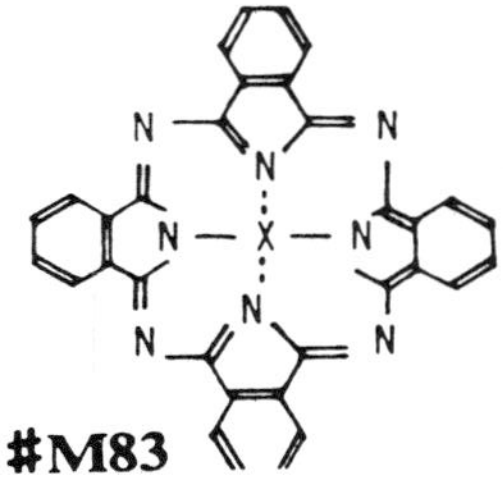

#M80— #M83

#M80 X = Mg
#M81 X = Zn
#M82 X = AlCl
#M83 X = GaCl

Table 12. Laser Characteristics of Xanthene Dyes[a]

Solvent	Concentration (mM)	Lasing wavelength (tuning) (nm)	Excitation	Output	Ref.
		#M84 Acridine red; acridine red 3B			
Ethanol	1	Orange (BB)	Ruby-SH (10 MW)		30
Ethanol	0.1	601.5 (BB)	Fl (50 J, 800 ns)	10 mJ	70
Ethanol	1	583.9 (BB)	N_2 (200 kW, 3ns, 10 Hz)	4 kW	71
Ethanol	2	578-598 (grating)	N_2 (10-20 kW, 10 ns)		72
Ethanol	2	619 (BB)	Ruby-SH (8 MW, 8 ns)	1.3 MW	73
		#M85 Pyronine Y; pyronine G			
Isoamyl alcohol		590 (BB)	Ruby and glass-SH		2
Isoamyl alcohol		585 (BB)	Fl		
Ethanol + HCl	0.1 g/l	590-653 (grating)	Fl (100 J, 800 ns, RT)		74

#M86 Pyronine B

Solvent	Conc.	Wavelength	Laser	Notes	Ref.
Methanol	1	Yellow (BB)	Fl (300 ns, RT)		75
Acetone or PMMA		576 (BB)	Glass-SH (18 MW)		76
Ethanol, PMMA, or glycerin	0.01		Glass-SH (2 MW, 40 ns)	$E \sim 30\%$	77
Ethanol		615–632 (BB, concentration)	Fl (0.5 μF, 20 kV, 750 ns, RT)		78
Ethanol	2	570–640 (grating)	Glass-SH (2 MW, 30 ns)	70 kW	79
Ethanol	0.2	599 (BB)	Fl (9 J, 80 ns, RT)	Thr = 0.7 J	1

#M87 Rhodamine C; rhodamine S

Solvent	Conc.	Wavelength	Laser	Notes	Ref.
Ethanol		570 (BB)	Glass-SH (8 MW) and -TH (1 MW)		76
Ethanol	0.2	598 (BB)	Fl (100 J, 1 μs, RT)	40 mJ	80
Ethanol, PMMA, or glycerin	0.01–1		Glass-SH (2 MW, 40 ns)	$E \sim 30\%$	77

(continued)

77

Table 12 *(continued)*

Solvent	Concentration (mM)	Lasing wavelength (tuning) (nm)	Excitation	Output	Ref.
Ethanol		578–594.5 (BB, concentration)	Fl (0.5 µF, 20 kV, 750 ns, RT)		78
Ethanol	0.2	600 (BB)	Fl (9 J, 80 ns, RT)	Thr = 0.7 J	1
Ethanol + DPB	0.15 + 4	622 (BB)	Fl (380 J, 30 µs)	300 mJ	81
#M88 Rhodamine 110; unsubstituted rhodamine; rhodamine 560; yellow 1					
		525–585 (prism)	Ar (488 nm		82
HFIP		540 (BB)	Fl		83
Trifluoro-ethanol		550 (BB)	Fl		
Ethanol (base)		560 (BB)	Fl		
Ethanol (acid)		570 (BB)	Fl		

Solvent	Conc.	Wavelength (nm)	Pump source	Output	Ref.
DMSO		575 (BB)	Fl		
EG	~3	536–603 (BF filter)	Ar (all lines, 4 W)	320 mW	35
Ethanol + DPB	0.06 + 2	570 (BB)	Fl (380 J, 30 μs)	185 mJ	81
		538–580 (BF filter + etalon) (ring cavity, single axial mode)	Ar (514 nm, 4 W)	830 mW	84
Polyurethanane	10	643 (DFB)	Ar (514 nm, 0.7 W)	0.1 μW	85
EG + COT	0.59 g/l	530–600 (BF filter + etalon)	Ar (all lines, 4 W)	280 mW	86
			Kr (blue-green, 2.3 W)	200 mW	
		532–590 (single axial mode)	AR (514 nm, 2.6 W)	160 mW	
Ethanol	3.33	547–592 (grating) (osc + amp)	XeCl (150 mJ, 10–20 ns)	E = 4.95%	26
Methanol		544–589 (grating)	Fl (150 ns, RT, 1 Hz)		87

(continued)

Table 12 (continued)

Solvent	Concentration (mM)	Lasing wavelength (tuning) (nm)	Excitation	Output	Ref.
EG + ammonyx LO + COT		530–582 (single axial mode, ring cavity)	Ar (all lines 23 W)	3.6 W	303
#M89 Rhodamine G					
Ethanol		585 (BB)	Ruby and glass–SH ($10\ MW/cm^2$)		88
Ethanol + DPB	0.1 + 5	616.5 (BB)	Fl (380 J, 30 μs)	300 mJ	81
#M90 Rhodamine B (chloride, perchlorate); N,N,N',N'-tetraethyl rhodamine; rhodamine 610; red 1; pilot 578					
Ethanol	2	608 (BB)	Ruby–SH (200 kW)		24
Methanol	1	Red (BB)	Fl (300 ns, RT)		75
Ethanol		577 (BB)	Ruby and glass–SH ($10\ MW/cm^2$)		88

Solvent		Wavelength	Pump	Output	Ref.
Ethanol	0.5	580–640 (grating)	Ruby-SH (5 MW, 15 ns)	300 kW	79
Ethanol + NaOH	0.5	586 (BB)	Glass-SH (2 MW, 30 ns)	120 kW	71
			N_2 (200 kW, 3 ns, 10 Hz)	2.6 kW	
Methanol	5	586–641 (prism + grating)	N_2 (130 kW)	19.1 kW	13
Ethanol (SA:DQTC) (SA:DODC)	0.15	605–639 (etalon) 615–645 (etalon)	Fl (1 kJ)	20 mJ (3–4 ps) mode locking	89
Water + 6 M acetamide	0.4	615–645 (etalon)	Fl (15 Hz, 450 Wav., 1.5 μs, RT)	128 mWav.	90
EG	~3	608–683 (BF filter)	Ar (all lines, 4W)	497 mW	35
		602–665 (BF filter + etalon) (ring cavity, single axial mode)	Ar (514 nm, 4 W)	680 mW	84

(continued)

Table 12 (*continued*)

Solvent	Concentration (mM)	Lasing wavelength (tuning) (nm)	Excitation	Output	Ref.
Ethanol + rhodamine 6G	0.15	621 (BB)	Fl (1.7 kJ, 1.7 µs)	1.7 J	91
Ethanol + NaOH	1.3	582–618 (grating) (osc + amp)	Cu (510 nm, 1.91 Wav., 6 kHz, 32 ns)	0.41 Wav. E = 20.7%	66
Ethanol		570–595 (grating) (osc + amp)	YAG–SH (100 mJ, 12 ns)	E = 26%	92
		600 (BB) (osc + amp)	Glass–SH (6 ps)	4 mJ, E = 12% (12 ps)	93
Ethanol	2	595–640 (grating)	YAG–TH (6–8 mJ, 8 ns)		94
Ethanol	2	619 (BB)	XeCl (60 mJ, 35 ns)	E = 27.2%	95

Solvent	Conc.	Tuning range	Pump	Output	Ref.
Ethanol	1	610–637 (BB) (ring cavity, injection lock)	Xe (2 kW, 250 ns, 5–10 Hz)	400 W beam	96
EG + COT	3.5 g/l	605–675 (BF filter + etalon)	Ar (all lines, 4 W)	500 mW, E = 13%	86
		605–660 (single axial mode)	Ar (514 nm, 2.6 W)	150 mW	
Ethanol	5	594–643 (grating) (osc + amp)	N_2 (1 MW, 10 ns, 50 Hz)	0.7 mJ	97
Ethanol	1.5	591–642 (grating) (osc + amp)	XeCl (150 mJ, 10–20 ns)	E = 7.8%	26

#M91 Rhodamine 3B

Solvent	Conc.	Tuning range	Pump	Output	Ref.
Isoamyl alcohol		620 (BB)	Ruby and glass–SH		2
		610 (BB)	Fl		
HFIP		610 (BB)	Fl		83
Trifluoro-ethanol		610 (BB)	Fl		

(continued)

Table 12 (continued)

Solvent	Concentration (mM)	Lasing wavelength (tuning) (nm)	Excitation	Output	Ref.
Ethanol		620 (BB)	Fl		
DMSO		630 (BB)	Fl		
Ethanol + DPB	0.15 + 4	631 (BB)	Fl (380 J, 30 μs)	360 mJ	81
Trifluoro-ethanol		623 (BB)	Fl (5 J)	1.7 mJ	67
#M92 Xylene red; xylene red B; kiton red S; kiton red 620; sulforhodamine B; red 2; acid red					
Ethanol (base)	50 mg/l	584–645 (grating)	Fl (0.3 μF, 25 kV, 500 ns, RT)		99
Ethanol (neutral)		589–642 (grating)			
Ethanol (base)	0.2	623 (BB)	Fl (9 J, 80 ns, RT)	Thr = 0.7 J	1
Methanol	0.1	600–655 (grating)	Fl (73 J)	350 mJ, (240 ns)	100

Solvent	Conc.	Tuning range (nm)	Pump	Output	Ref.
Methanol		605–625 (prism) (ring cavity, single axial mode)	Fl (60 J)	1 kW	101
EG	~3	610–680 (BF filter)	Ar (all lines, 4 W)		35
Trifluoro-ethanol	1.7	595–639 (grating) (osc + amp)	Cu (510 and 578 nm, 4.03 Wav., 32 ns, 6 kHz)	0.76 Wav., $E = 18.2\%$	66
Trifluoro-ethanol		603–648 (grating)	N_2 (2 mJ, 8 ns, 5 Hz)	38 μJ	67
		629 (BB)	Fl (5 J)	1.8 mJ	
		570–605 (grating) (osc + amp)	YAG-SH (200 mJ)	$E = 29\%$	98
Ethanol	1.25	590–645 (grating) (osc + amp)	XeCl (150 mJ, 10–20 ns)	$E = 9.9\%$	26

#M93 Lissamine rhodamine B-200; sulforhodamine B monosodium salt

Solvent	Conc.	Tuning range (nm)	Pump	Output	Ref.
Ethanol	100 mg/1	575–635 (grating)	Fl (100 J, 800 ns, RT)		74

(continued)

Table 12 (continued)

Solvent	Concentration (mM)	Lasing wavelength (tuning) (nm)	Excitation	Output	Ref.
#M94 Rhodamine 6G (chloride, perchlorate, tetrafluoroborate); rhodamine 590; orange 1; pilot 559					
Ethanol	0.03–3	Green to orange (BB)	Ruby-SH (10 MW)	Thr = 100–200 kW	30
Ethanol	~0.1	585 (BB)	Fl (50 J, 800 ns)	70 mJ	70
Methanol	1	Orange-yellow (BB)	Fl (300 ns, RT)		75
Ethanol	2×10^{15} cm^{-3}	565 (BB)	Ruby and glass-SH (10 MW/cm^2)	12 mJ (15 ns)	88
Ethanol	0.1	595–616 (grating)	Fl (50 J)	200 mJ	102
PMMA	0.14	601 (BB)	Fl (200 J)		103
Alcohol	1	(BB)	N$_2$ (83 kW, 10 ns, 70 Hz)	E = 25%	104
		565–620	N$_2$ (120 kW, 10 ns,	E = 22%	130

86

Solvent	Conc.	Wavelength	Pump	Output	Ref.
Ethanol + COT	0.05	~600 (BB)	Fl (524 J, 650 μs)	160 mJ (600 μs, long pulse)	105
Water + 1.5% triton X-100	0.25	597 (BB)	Ar (514 nm, 960 mW)	30 mW	106
Water + 4% ammonyx LO	0.4	560–655 (prism)	Ar (514 nm, 3.5 W)	1 W, E = 30%	107
Water + 5% ammonyx LO	0.5	570 (BB)	Xe (300 W, 450 ns, 120 Hz)	12 W, 300 ns	108
Water + 4% triton X-100	1	590 (BB)	Spark in Ar (600 ns, 0.1 J, 500 Hz)	60 W_{peak}	109
Methanol + COT	0.4	(BB)	Fl (1 kJ, 5 μs)	12 J, E = 1.2%	110
Ethanol	0.022	(BB)	Fl (50 kJ, 25 μs)	400 J (10 μs)	111
	0.25	(BB)	Fl (211 J, 350 Hz)	114 Wav. (at 250 Hz)	112

(continued)

Table 12 (continued)

Solvent	Concentration (mM)	Lasing wavelength (tuning) (nm)	Excitation	Output	Ref.
Ethanol	0.2	(BB)	Fl (34 kWav., 17 μs, 50 Hz)	109 Wav., E = 0.32%	113
Ethanol	2	600 (BB)	Argon-jet spark (150 mJ, 100 Hz)	1 mWav. (200 W, 50 ns)	114
Methanol	1–30	590–610 (BB, concentration)	CO_2-laser-produced plasma (5.6 J)	2 mJ (70 ns)	115
Ethanol	0.125 g/l	(grating + etalon) (osc + amp) (single axial mode)	Xe (3.2 mJ, 160 ns, 30 Hz)	0.2 mJ (100 ns)	116
EG	3	570–655 (BF filter)	Ar (all lines, 4 W)	0.9 W	35
Water + 18% ammonyx LO + 1.3% PVA		(BB)	Ar (all lines, 110 W)	33 W	117
			Ar (all lines, 175 W)	52 W	

MBBA (liquid crystal)	1	602-623 (BB, temperature)	N_2		118
Ethanol	1	564-600 (grating) (osc + amp)	Cu (510 nm, 2.1 Wav., 32 ns, 6 kHz)	0.65 Wav., E = 29.7%	66
PMMA	1-10	555-565 (BB)	CdS (e-beam pumped, 495 nm, 15 ns, 15 W_{peak}, 1 kHz, 77 K)	0.3 W_{peak} E = 2%	119
Ethanol		550-590 (grating) (osc + amp)	YAG-SH (100 mJ, 12 ns, 20 Hz)	35 mJ, E = 35%	92
Ethanol	1	580 (BB)	KrF (0.2 J, 20 ns)	E = 5%	120
Ethanol	4	591 (BB)	XeCl (60 mJ, 35 ns)	E = 27.7%	95
Ethanol (SA:DODC)	0.125	584-625 (etalon)	Fl (1 kJ)	40 mJ (2.5 ps) mode locking	89
EG (SA: DODC)		(BB)	Ar (514 nm, 2.5 W)	4 kW/pulse (0.5-1 ps) mode locking, cavity dumping	121

(continued)

Table 12 *(continued)*

Solvent	Concentration (mM)	Lasing wavelength (tuning) (nm)	Excitation	Output	Ref.
EG (SA:DODC)		565–630 (BF filter + etalon) (ring cavity, single axial mode)	Ar (514 nm, 9 W)	2.2 W	84
EG	0.59 g/l	560–650 (BF filter + etalon)	Ar (all lines, 4 W)	1 W, E = 25%	86
		560–650 (BF filter + etalon)	Kr (blue–green, 2.3 W)	0.7 W, E = 33%	
		565–635 (single axial mode)	Ar (514 nm, 2.5 W)	220 mW	
Ethanol	5	568–605 (grating) (osc + amp)	N_2 (1 MW, 10 ns, 50 Hz)	0.8 mJ	97

Solvent	Conc.	Tuning range (nm)	Pump	Efficiency/Output	Ref.
Ethanol	2.5	570–616 (grating) (osc + amp)	XeCl (150 nm, 10–20 ns)	E = 15.1%	26
		550–620	Cu (510 nm, 75 kW, 25 ns, 6 kHz)	E = 57%	50
EG + ammonyx LO + COT		572–620 (single axial mode, ring cavity)	Ar (all lines, 24 W)	5.6 W	303

#M95 Rhodamine 19; rhodamine 575; yellow 2

Solvent	Conc.	Tuning range (nm)	Pump	Efficiency/Output	Ref.
Ethanol (base)		575 (BB)	Fl		83
Ethanol (acid)		585 (BB)	Fl		
Ethanol		563–602 (grating)	Fl (150 ns, RT, 1 Hz)		87

#M96 Rhodamine derivative 1; *N,N'*-bispentamethylene rhodamine

Solvent	Conc.	Tuning range (nm)	Pump	Efficiency/Output	Ref.
Ethanol		598 (BB)	Glass–SH		122

#M97 Rhodamine derivative 2; *N,N'*-di-β-phenylethyl rhodamine

Solvent	Conc.	Tuning range (nm)	Pump	Efficiency/Output	Ref.
Ethanol		559 (BB)	Glass–SH		122

(continued)

Table 12 (continued)

Solvent	Concentration (mM)	Lasing wavelength (tuning) (nm)	Excitation	Output	Ref.
Ethanol + water (1:1)	0.3	571–615 (prism)	Ar (514 nm, 0.7 W)	40 mW	123
Ethanol	(0.9–1.3) $\times 10^{17}$ cm^{-3}	565 (BB)	Glass–SH		124
#M98 Rhodamine derivative 3; N,N'-bis(butyl)rhodamine					
Ethanol + DPB	0.2 + 20	598 (BB)	Fl (380 J, 30 μs)	150 mJ	81
#M99 Rhodamine derivative 4; N,N'-bis(methyl-butyl)rhodamine					
Ethanol + DPB	0.2 + 5	625 (BB)	Fl (380 J, 30 μs)	105 mJ	81
Ethanol + DPB	0.02 + 5	612 (BB)	Fl (380 J, 30 μs)	17 mJ	81
#M100 Rhodamine derivative 5; N,N'-diethyl rhodamine					
Ethanol	(0.9 – 1.3) $\times 10^{17}$ cm^{-3}	568 (BB)	Glass–SH		124

Ethanol + DPB	0.15 + 2	596.5 (BB)	Fl (380 J, 30 μs)	400 mJ	81

#M101 Rhodamine derivative 6; *N,N'*-dibutylrhodamine

Ethanol + DPB	0.2 + 2	590 (BB)	Fl (380 J, 30 μs)	240 mJ	81

#M102 Rhodamine derivative 7

Ethanol	$(0.9-1.3) \times 10^{17}$ cm^{-3}	572 (BB)	Glass-SH		124

#M103 Rhodamine derivative 8; *N,N'*-dibenzylrhodamine

Ethanol	$(0.9-1.3) \times 10^{17}$ cm^{-3}	546 (BB)	Glass-SH		124

Ethanol + DPB	0.2 + 20	583 (BB)	Fl (380 J, 30 μs)	122 mJ	81

#M104 Rhodamine derivative 9

Ethanol	$(0.9-1.3) \times 10^{17}$ cm^{-3}	518 (BB)	Glass-SH		124

#M105 Rhodamine derivative 10

Ethanol	$(0.9-1.3) \times 10^{17}$ cm^{-3}	510 (BB)	Glass-SH		124

(continued)

Table 12 *(continued)*

Solvent	Concentration (mM)	Lasing wavelength (tuning) (nm)	Excitation	Output	Ref.
#M106 Rhodamine derivative 11					
Ethanol	$(0.9-1.3) \times 10^{17}$ cm^{-3}	599 (BB)	Glass-SH		124
#M107 Rhodamine derivative 12					
Ethanol	$(0.9-1.3) \times 10^{17}$ cm^{-3}	617 (BB)	Glass-SH		124
#M108 Rhodamine 5G					
Ethanol + DPB	0.15 + 4	599.5 (BB)	Fl (380 J, 30 μs)	400 mJ	81
#M109 Rhodamine 101; rhodamine 640; red 3					
HFIP		625 (BB)	Fl		83
Trifluoro-ethanol		625 (BB)	Fl		

Solvent	Conc.	Wavelength (nm)	Pump	Output	Efficiency (%)
Ethanol (base)		630 (BB)	Fl		
Ethanol (acid)		640 (BB)	Fl		
DMSO		650 (BB)	Fl		
Ethanol		590–620 (grating) (osc + amp)	YAG-SH (100 mJ, 12 ns)	22 mJ, E = 22%	92
Methanol + water (3:2)	3.5	620–680 (grating)	YAG-TH (6–8 mJ, 8 ns)		94
DMSO + HCl		630–700 (grating)	N_2 (2 mJ, 8 ns, 5 Hz)	55 µJ	67
+ rhodamine 6G		620–675 (BF filter + etalon) (ring cavity, single axial mode)	Ar (514 nm, 4 W)	660 mW	84
Methanol	0.12	(prism)	Fl (750 J)	4 J, E = 0.53%	125
EG	1.76 g/l	615–695 (BF filter + etalon)	Ar (all lines, 4 W)	430 mW	86

(continued)

Table 12 (continued)

Solvent	Concentration (mM)	Lasing wavelength (tuning) (nm)	Excitation	Output	Ref.
EG	0.88 g/l	615–710 (BF filter + etalon)	Kr (blue–green, 2.5 W)	510 mW	
EG	0.88 g/l	620–690 (single axial mode)	Kr (blue–green, 2.5 W)	65 mW	
Ethanol	1.2	613–672 (grating) (osc + amp)	XeCl (150 mJ, 10–20 ns)	E = 11.2%	26
Methanol		620–670 (grating)	Fl (10 Hz)	0.9 Wav. (1.4 μs)	126
Methanol		610–690	Cu (510 nm, 578 nm, 100 kW, 25 ns, 6 kHz)	E = 52%	50
Methanol		590–620 (grating) (osc + amp)	YAG–SH (200 mJ)	E = 26%	98

Solvent	Conc.	Wavelength (nm)	Pump	Output	
DMSO		600–630 (grating) (osc + amp)	YAG-SH (200 mJ)	E = 26%	

#M110 Sulforhodamine 101; sulforhodamine 640

Solvent	Conc.	Wavelength (nm)	Pump	Output	Ref.
Methanol + water (1:1)	0.50 g/l	656 (BF filter)	Ar (514 nm, 1.8 W)	40 mW	127
Ethanol (acid)	0.15	590–640 (prism)	YAG-SH (24 MW, 10 ns, 10 Hz)	9 MW (10 ns)	128
EG	2.14	644–686 (BF filter)	Ar (all lines, 3.2 W)	55 mW	129
EG + rhodamine 6G	3 + 1	641–694 (BF filter)	Ar (all lines, 3.2 W)	88 mW	
Methanol + water		630–690 (grating)	Fl (10 Hz)	0.9 Wav. (1.3 µs)	126

#M111 Rhodamine 6Y

Solvent		Wavelength (nm)	Pump		Ref.
Ethanol		572 (BB)	Glass-SH		122

#M112 Fluorescein (Na salt, K salt); disodiumfluorescein; uranine

Solvent	Conc.	Wavelength (nm)	Pump		Ref.
Water + NaOH	10	539 (BB)	Ruby-SH (200 kW)		24

(continued)

97

Table 12 (continued)

Solvent	Concentration (mM)	Lasing wavelength (tuning) (nm)	Excitation	Output	Ref.
Water	1	Green	Ruby–SH (10 MW)		30
Ethanol	1	Green	Ruby–SH (10 MW)		
Ethanol	0.1	550 (BB)	Fl (50 J, 800 ns)	1 mJ	70
Alcohol	0.5	(BB)	N_2 (83 kW, 10 ns, 45 Hz)	E = 11%	104
		520–600 (grating)	N_2 (120 kW, 10 ns, 100 Hz)	E = 20% (4 ns)	130
Water	0.3	530–570 (grating)	Ruby–SH (5 MW, 15 ns)	20 kW	79
Ethanol	1	540–580 (grating)	Ruby–SH (5 MW, 15 ns)	100 kW	
Ethanol	1	542–580 (grating)	Glass–SH (2 MW, 30 ns)	40 kW	
Methanol	5	528–564 (prism + grating)	N_2 (130 kW)	29.3 kW	13

Solvent	Conc.	Wavelength	Pump	Power	Ref.
Water + ammonyx LO + COT + NaOH	0.2	522–570 (prism)	Ar (all lines, 2 W)	70 mW	131
Methanol + COT + Na_2CO_3	0.3	549–574 (grating)	Fl (11 J, 1 μs)	2 kW, E = 1%	132
EG	3	536–581 (BF filter)	Ar (all lines, 4 W)	386 mW	35
Ethanol + DPB	0.2 + 7	561 (BB)	Fl (380 J, 30 μs)	53 mJ	81
Ethanol	0.2	531 (BB) K salt	N_2 (1 MW, 10 ns)		133
Ethanol + COT	0.4	550–565 (etalon)	Fl (15 Hz, 450 Wav., 1.5 μs, RT)	25 mWav.	90
Ethanol	4	550 (BB)	XeCl (60 mJ, 35 ns)	E = 7.6%	95
EG + COT	1.76 g/l	540–580 (BF filter + etalon)	Ar (all lines, 4 W)	0.5 W	86

#M113 Monobromofluorescein

| Glycerin | | 560 (BB) | Ruby-SH | | 2 |

(continued)

Table 12 *(continued)*

Solvent	Concentration (mM)	Lasing wavelength (tuning) (nm)	Excitation	Output	Ref.
#M114 2',7'-Dichlorofluorescein					
Ethanol			Fl (50 J, 800 ns)		102
Ethanol + NaOH	0.3	544.2 (BB)	N_2 (200 kW, 3 ns, 10 Hz)	3.7 kW	71
Ethanol (base) + anthracene		575 (BB)	Ar (515 nm)	Thr = 0.33 W	134
Methanol + COT + Na_2CO_3	0.5	557–581 (grating)	Fl (11 J, 1 μs)	2.6 kW (0.6 μs)	132
Ethanol	10	541–583 (grating + prism)	N_2 (130 kW)	24.5 kW	13
#M115 4',5'-Dibromofluorescein					
Glycerin		568 (BB)	Ruby-SH		2

		#M116 2',4',5',7'-Tetrachlorofluorescein			
Ethanol (base) + anthracene	20	582 (BB)	Ar (515 nm)	Thr = 1.1 W	134
			Fl	Thr = 36 J	
#M117 2',4',5',7'-Tetrabromofluorescein; eosin; eosin Y					
Ethanol	1	Yellow	Ruby-SH (10 MW)		30
Methanol (base)		553–557	Ruby and glass-SH		52
Ethanol + NaOH	0.5	558.2	N_2 (200 kW, 3 ns, 10 Hz)	0.35 kW	71
DMF	0.5	570.5	N_2 (200 kW, 3 ns, 10 Hz)	0.4 kW	
#M118 6-Carboxyfluorescein					
Ethanol + NaOH	30 mg/l	539–548 (BB)	Fl (200 J, 800 ns, RT)		74
#M119 Fluorescein isothiocyanate					
Ethanol (base)	0.2	546 (BB)	Fl (9 J, 80 ns, RT)	Thr = 6.2 J	1

(continued)

Table 12 (continued)

Solvent	Concentration (mM)	Lasing wavelength (tuning) (nm)	Excitation	Output	Ref.
#M120 Fluorescein diacetate; diacetylfluorescein					
Ethanol (base)	50 mg/l	541–571 (BB)	Fl (0.3 μF, 25 kV, 500 ns, RT)		99
Ethanol + NaOH	40 mg/l		Fl (200 J, 800 ns, RT)		74
#M121 Chromogen red B					
Methanol + NaOH		565–585 (grating)	N$_2$ (1 mJ, 8 ns, 5 Hz)	1.7 μJ	135
		570–598 (grating)	Coumarin dye laser (480 nm, 0.1 mJ, 6 ns)	2 μJ	
#M122 Naphthofluorescein 126					
Ethanol (base)		700 (BB)	Fl		60

[a] Structures.

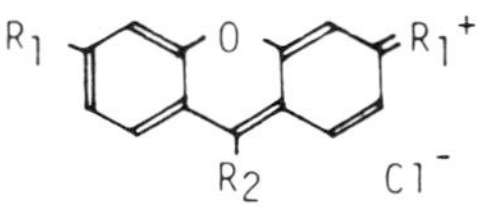

#M84* $R_1 = NHMe$, $R_2 = H$
#M85 $R_1 = NMe_2$, $R_2 = H$
#M86 $R_1 = NEt_2$, $R_2 = H$
#M87 $R_1 = NMe_2$, $R_2 = C_2H_4COOH$

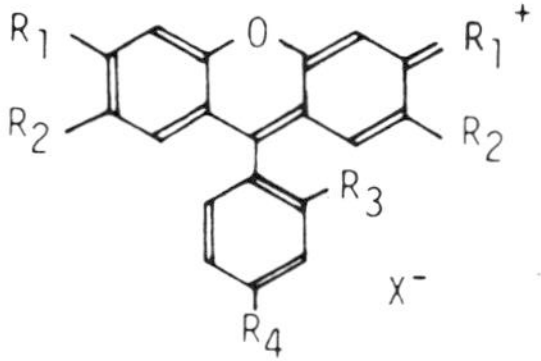

#M88— #M108

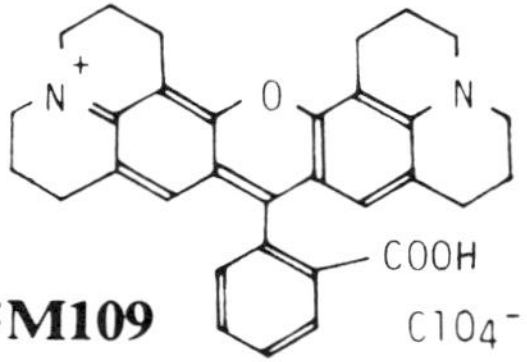

#M109

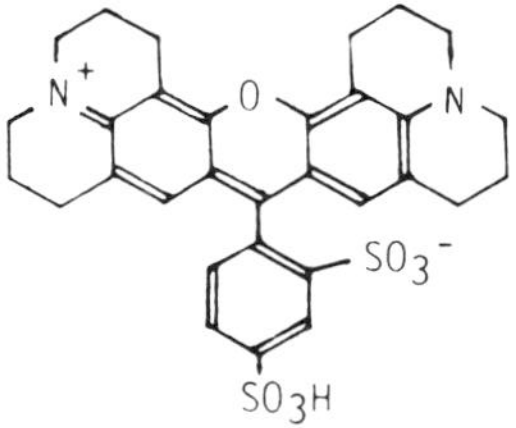

#M110

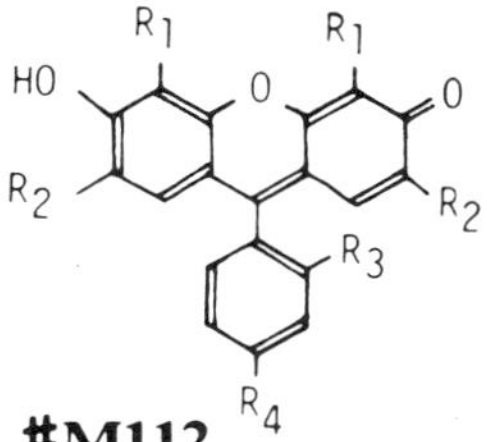

#M112,
#M114— #M118

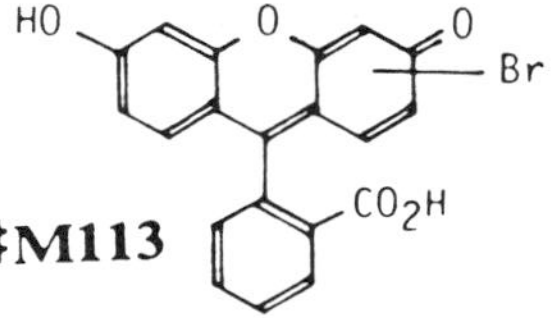

#M113

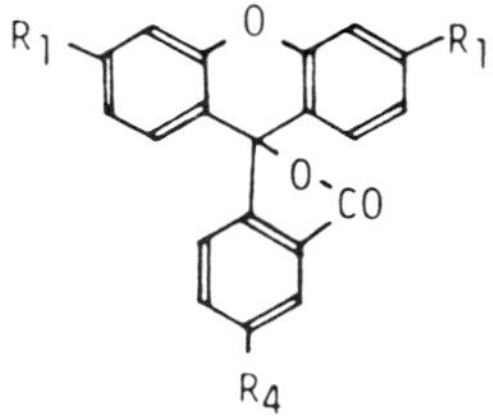

#M119, #M120

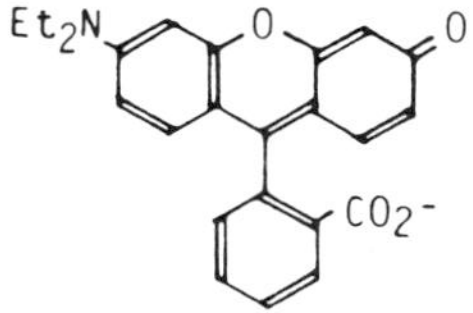

#M121

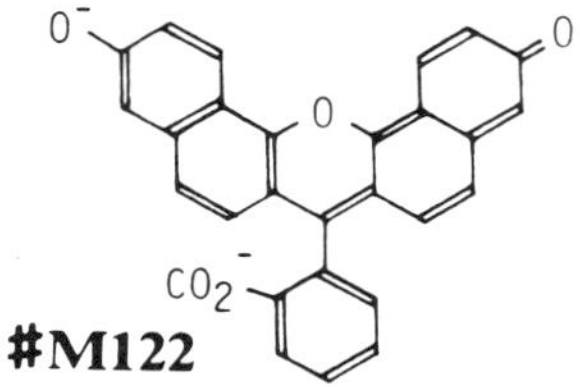

#M122

(continued)

Table 12 (continued)

Dye no.	R_1	R_2	R_3	R_4	X
#M88	NH_2	H	COOH	H	Cl
#M89	NHEt	H	COOH	H	Cl
#M90	NEt_2	H	COOH	H	Cl, ClO_4
#M91	NEt_2	H	COOEt	H	ClO_4
#M92	NEt_2	H	SO_3^-	SO_3H	—
#M93	NEt_2	H	SO_3^-	SO_3Na	—
#M94	NHEt	Me	COOEt	H	Cl, ClO_4, BF_4
#M95	NHEt	Me	COOH	H	ClO_4
#M96	N-piperidinyl	H	COOH	H	X
#M97	NHC_2H_4Ph	H	COOH	H	X
#M98*	NBu_2	H	COOH	H	X
#M99*	NMeBu	H	COOH	H	X
#M100	NHEt	H	COOH	H	X
#M101*	NHBu	H	COOH	H	X
#M102	NHEt	H	COOEt	H	X

104

#					
#M103	NHCH$_2$Ph	H	COOH	H	X
#M104	NC$_4$H$_8$	H	COOH	H	X
#M105	NC$_6$H$_{12}$	H	COOH	H	X
#M106	NHPh + NHC$_2$H$_4$Ph	H	COOH	H	X
#M107	NHPh + NHC$_3$H$_9$Ph	H	COOH	H	X
#M108	NHMe	Me	Cl	H	X
#M112	H	H	COOH	H	—
#M114	H	Cl	COOH	H	—
#M115	Br	H	COOH	H	—
#M116	Cl	Cl	COOH	H	—
#M117	Br	Br	COOH	H	—
#M118	H	H	COOH	COOH	—
#M119	OH	—	—	NCS	—
#M120	CH$_3$COO	—	—	H	—

*Estimated structure.

Table 13.   Laser Characteristics of Triarylmethane Dyes[a]

Solvent	Lasing wavelength (tuning) (nm)	Excitation	Ref.
	#M123 Brilliant green		
Glycerin	759 (BB)	Ruby	2
	#M124 Rhoduline blue 6G		
Glycerin	758 (BB)	Ruby	2
	#M125 Victoria blue R		
Glycerin	814 (BB)	Ruby	2
	#M126 Victoria blue		
Glycerin	809 (BB)	Ruby	2
	#M127 Naphthalene green		
Glycerin	756 (BB)	Ruby	2

[a] Estimated structures:

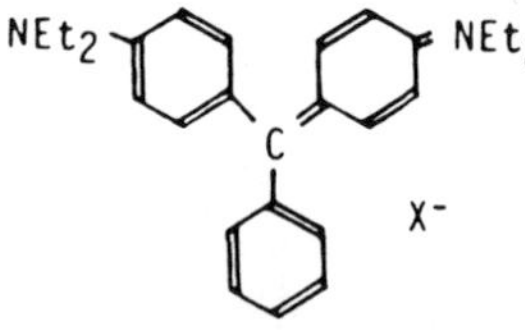

#M123*

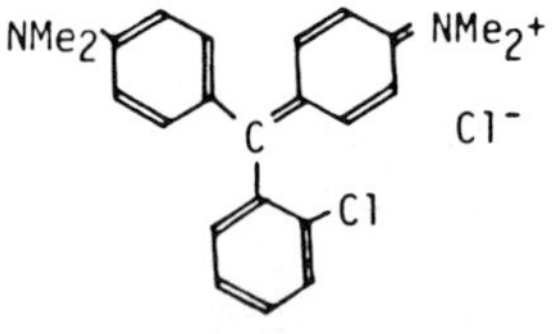

#M124

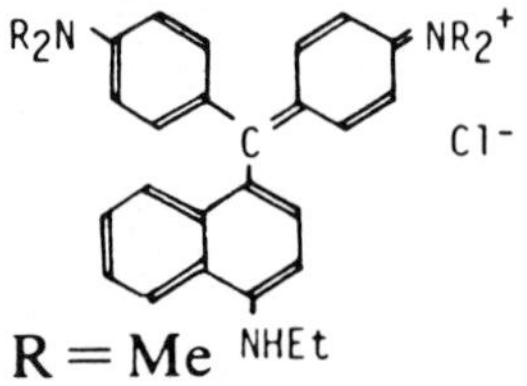

#M125* R = Me   NHEt
#M126* R = Et

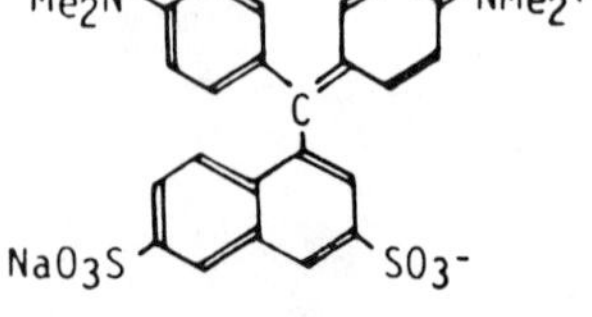

#M127*

Table 14. Laser Characteristics of Acridine Dyes[a]

Solvent	Concentration (mM)	Lasing wavelength (tuning) (nm)	Excitation	Output	Ref.
		#M128 Acridine yellow			
Ethanol	0.2	514 (BB)	Fl (9 J, 80 ns, RT)		1
		#M129 9-Aminoacridine hydrochloride			
Ethanol or water (acid)		457-460 (BB)	Fl (0.5 µF, 20 kV, 750 ns, RT)		78
Methanol		449-453	Fl		52
Ethanol	1	458 (BB)	Fl (9 J, 80 ns, RT)	Thr = 1.1 J	1
		#M130 *N*-Methylacridinium perchlorate			
Methyl cellosolve	10	535-553 (BB)	N_2 (100 kW, 10 ns)		136

(continued)

Table 14 (continued)

Solvent	Concentration (mM)	Lasing wavelength (tuning) (nm)	Excitation	Output	Ref.
		#M131 Acriflavine; trypaflavine			
Ethanol		510 (BB)	Ruby-SH (10 MW/cm^2)		88
Ethanol	36	517.4 (BB)	Fl (20 J, 50 ns, RT)	Thr = 7.4 J	137
Ethanol + DAMC (9:50)	5	494-528 (prism + grating)	N$_2$ (130 kW)	13 kW	13
		#M132 Lucigenin			
Water + H$_2$SO$_4$		600 (BB)	Ruby-SH		2
		#M133 9-(10H)acridone			
Ethanol	>1	438.5 (BB)	Ruby-SH (10 MW)		30
Ethanol		435 (BB)	Fl (90 J, 100 ns, RT)	20.3 kW	138
Ethanol	5	436 (BB)	N$_2$ (530 kW, 3.5 ns)	E = 3.6%	139

#M134 Carbazine 122; carbazine 720; red 7

Solvent		Wavelength	Pump	Conditions	Ref.
Ethanol (base)		720 (BB)	Fl		60
DMSO (base)		740 (BB)	Fl		
Ethanol + NaOH	0.4	700 (BB)	YAG-SH (24 MW)	10.5 MW, E = 44%	140
Water + ammonyx LO (base)		670–727 (etalon)	Mode-locked YAG-SH (0.9 mJ/pulse, 30 ps)	(12 ps) (synchronous pumping)	141
Ethanol (base)		660–710 (grating) (osc + amp)	YAG-SH (100 mJ, 12 ns)	18 mJ, E = 18%	92
		670–750	Cu (578 nm, 25 kW, 25 ns, 6 kHz)	E = 35%	50
		684–730 (grating) (osc + amp)	YAG-SH (200 mJ)	E = 13%	98
EG + ethanol (base)		687–811 (BF filter)	Kr (647, 676 nm)		298

(continued)

109

Table 14 *(continued)*

[a]Structures:

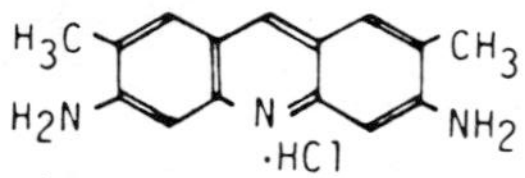

#M128

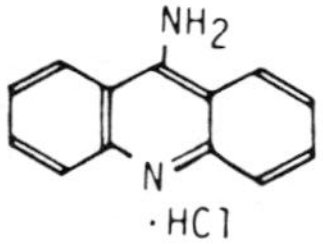

#M129

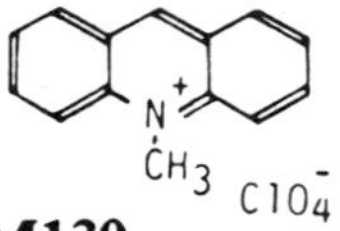

#M130

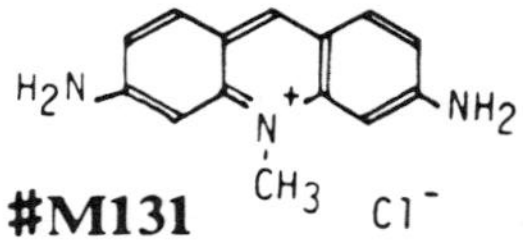

#M131

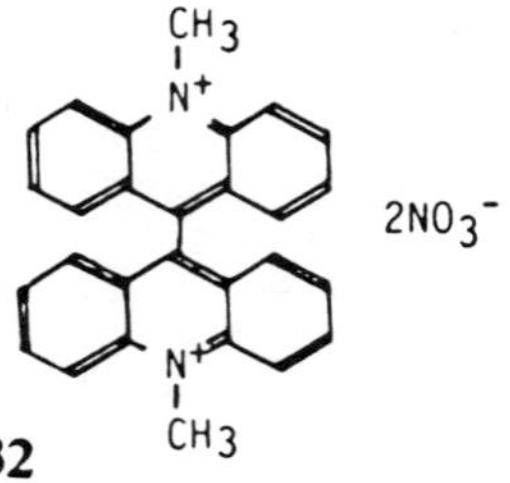

#M132

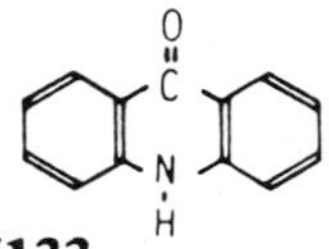

#M133

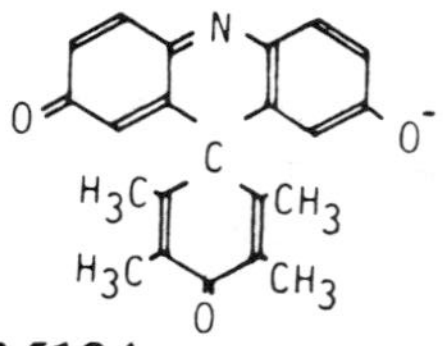

#M134

110

Table 15. Laser Characteristics of Azine Dyes[a]

Solvent	Concentration (mM)	Lasing wavelength (tuning) (nm)	Excitation	Output	Ref.
		#M135 Oxazine 118			
Ethanol		630 (BB)	Laser pumping (pulse)		83
	#M136 Oxazine 1,oxazine 725; pilot 740				
Ethanol		715 (BB)	Laser pumping (pulse)		83
Trifluorotoluene		730 (BB)	Fl		
EG	~3	690–780 (BF filter)	Kr (647 nm, 0.75 W)		35
Methanol + rhodamine 6G	0.08 + 0.1	705–745 (grating)	Fl (86 J)	25 mJ	100
Dichloromethane	0.4	690 (BB)	YAG-SH (24 MW, 10 ns, 10 Hz)	550 mWav., E = 23%	36
Glycerin + DMSO (1:1)	1.1	684–796 (BF filter)	Kr (647 and 676 nm, 5 W)	1.3 W	18

(continued)

111

Table 15 (continued)

Solvent	Concentration (mM)	Lasing wavelength (tuning) (nm)	Excitation	Output	Ref.
DMSO + EG (1:3)	1	685–825 (BF filter)	Mode locked Kr (647 nm, 1.4 W, 200 ps)	420 mWav. (~25 ps) (syn-chronous pumping)	39
DMSO + EG (1:6) + (SA: hex-acyanine 3)	1	700 (BF filter)	Mode locked Kr (647 nm, 1.1 W, 100 ps)	120 mWav. (6.7 ps) 120 mWav. (0.35 ps)	142
Methylene chloride	0.04	688.5 (etalon)	Fl Rhodamine B laser (620 nm, 130 mJ, 200 ns)	E = 20%	19
		695–770 (BF filter + etalon) (ring cavity, single axial mode)	Kr (647 and 676 nm, 5.5 W)	1 W	84

Solvent	Conc.	Tuning range (nm)	Pump	Output	Ref.
Ethanol	2.1	692–768 (grating) (osc + amp)	XeCl (150 mJ, 10–20 ns)	E = 5.6%	26
EG	1.2 g/l	695–800 (BF filter + etalon)	Kr (647 and 676 nm, 4 W)	1.3 W, E = 30–35%	86
EG	1.2 g/l	695–800 (single axial mode)	Kr (647 and 676 nm, 2.5 W)	200 mW	
Ethanol + rhodamine B	5 + 5	705–750 (grating) (osc + amp)	N_2 (1 MW, 10 ns, 50 Hz)	0.25 mJ	97
Dichloromethane		720–758 (grating)	Fl (150 ns, RT, 1 Hz)		87
		700–760	Cu (510 and 578 nm, 100 kW, 25 ns, 6 kHz)	E = 20%	50

#M137 Oxazine 4

| Ethanol | | 650 (BB) | Laser pumping (pulse) | | 83 |

#M138 Oxazine 170; oxazine 720; red 6[b]

| Methanol | | 690–740 | Fl | | 143 |

(continued)

Table 15 *(continued)*

Solvent	Concentration (mM)	Lasing wavelength (tuning) (nm)	Excitation	Output	Ref.
Ethanol + sulfo-rhodamine 101	0.4	672 (BB)	YAG-SH (24 MW, 10 ns, 10 Hz)	430 mWav.	36
Ethanol	1.5	664–690 (grating)	YAG-TH (6–8 mJ, 8 ns)		94
Methanol		680–710 (grating)	Fl (10 Hz)	0.7 Wav. (1.4 µs)	126
Methanol		650–700 (grating) (osc + amp)	YAG-SH (200 mJ)	E = 10%	98

#M139 Nile blue A (perchlorate, nitrate); nile blue 690; red 5; pilot 730

Solvent	Concentration (mM)	Lasing wavelength (tuning) (nm)	Excitation	Output	Ref.
Methanol			Mode-locked HeNe (intracavity pump)		145
Methanol + rhodamine 6G	0.75 + 0.05	690–745 (grating) nitrate	Fl (86 J)	50 mJ (240 ns)	100

114

Solvent	Conc.	Output range (nm)	Excitation source	Power/Energy	No.
EG	~3	692–784 (BF filter)	Kr (647 nm, 0.75 W)	70 mW	35
EG		720 (BB)	Rhodamine 6G CW laser (582.5 nm) (Ar at 514 nm, 9 W)	200 mW	144
Methanol	0.2	683 (BB)	Cresyl violet laser (647 nm, 11 MW, 10 Hz)	460 mWav., E = 42%	36
Glycerin + DMSO (1:4)		690–796 (BF filter)	Kr (647 and 676 nm, 5 W)	500 mW	18
Ethanol	1	710 (BB)	XeCl (60 mJ, 35 ns)	E = 12.6%	95
			N_2 (3.5 mJ, 14 ns)	E = 8.2%	
Methanol + water (3:2) + rhodamine 640	1.5 + 0.15	682–715 (grating)	YAG-TH (6–8 mJ, 8 ns)		94
Ethanol + rhodamine B	0.8 + 3.8	683–710 (grating) (osc + amp)	N_2 (1 MW, 50 Hz, 10 ns)	0.33 mJ	83
Ethanol	2	683–705 (grating) (osc + amp)	XeCl (150 mJ, 10–20 ns)	E = 1.3%	26

(continued)

Table 15 (continued)

Solvent	Concentration (mM)	Lasing wavelength (tuning) (nm)	Excitation	Output	Ref.
#M140 Cresyl violet (choride, perchlorate, acetate, nitrate); oxazine 9; cresyl violet 670; red 4					
Ethanol	100 mg/l	646–709 (grating)	Fl (100 J, 800 ns, RT)		74
Ethanol	2	643–660 (grating)	N_2 (10–20 kW, 10 ns)		72
Methanol	0.15–0.24	650	Mode-locked HeNe (intracavity pump)	0.6 mW	145
Ethanol + rhodamine B	Satur + 5 (5:300)	625–654 (grating + prism) acetate	N_2 (130 kW)	10.6 kW	13
	(25:300)	634–667		6.6 kW	
+ rhodamine B		612–697 (grating, concentration) acetate	N_2 (250 kW)	> 10 kW	14

Ethanol + rhodamine 6G	0.05 + 0.2	655 (BB)	Ruby-SH (8 MW, 8 ns)	0.5 MW	73
Ethanol + rhodamine 6G + (SA:DTDC)	0.14	652–704 (etalon)	Fl (1 kJ)	10–20 mJ (mode locked, 3 ps)	89
+ (SA:DDC or DOTC)		644–680 (etalon)			
Methanol	0.4	660–685 (etalon)	Fl (15 Hz, 450 Wav., 1.5 µs, RT)	112 mWav.	90
+ rhodamine 6G	0.4 + 0.2			187 mWav.	
Ethanol	0.24 g/l	660 (BB)	Xe (300 W, 450 ns, 120 Hz)	20 W_{peak} (300 ns)	108
Methanol		645–700 (prism + etalon) (single axial mode)	Fl (60 J)	0.8 kW	101
Methanol + rhodamine 6G	0.02 + 0.05	630–690 (grating) acetate	Fl (73 J)	210 mJ (240 ns)	100

(continued)

117

Table 15 (continued)

Solvent	Concentration (mM)	Lasing wavelength (tuning) (nm)	Excitation	Output	Ref.
Methanol + rhodamine 6G	0.08 + 0.05	645–705 (grating) nitrate	Fl (73 J)	290 mJ (240 ns)	100
EG	~3	650–697 (BF filter)	Ar (all lines, 5 W)	200 mW	35
EG		690 (BB)	Rhodamine 6G CW laser (582.5 nm) (Ar at 514 nm, 9 W)	585 mW	144
Ethanol + rhodamine 6G	0.15	686 (BB)	Fl (1.7 kJ, 1.7 μs)	1.1 J	91
Methanol	2	653–663 (grating)	N_2 (100 kW)	E = 0.2%	146
		622 (BB)	Rhodamine 6G laser (10 kW, 5 ns)	E = 10%	
Methanol + water	0.25	620–670 (prism)	YAG-SH (24 MW, 10 ns, 10 Hz)	8 MW	128

Solvent	Conc.	Tuning range	Pump	Output	Ref.
Methanol		620–671 (etalon)	Mode-locked YAG-SH (0.9 mJ, 30 ps) (synchronous pumping)		141
Ethanol	Satur.	659.4 (BB)	XeCl (60 mJ, 35 ns)	$E = 21.5\%$	95
Ethanol	2	651–701 (grating) (osc + amp)	XeCl (150 mJ, 10–20 ns)	$E = 6.8\%$	26
Ethanol + rhodamine 6G	3.3 + 2.5	641–687 (grating) (osc + amp)	N_2 (1 MW, 10 ns, 50 Hz)	0.38 mJ	97
+ rhodamine B	0.6 + 2.5	628–651 (grating) (osc + amp)	N_2 (1 MW, 10 ns, 50 Hz)	0.4 mJ	
		620–670 (grating) (osc + amp)	YAG-SH (200 mJ)	$E = 16\%$	98

#M141 Nile blue A oxazone; phenoxasone 9

Solvent	Conc.	Tuning range	Pump	Output	Ref.
Ether	1	580–631 (BF filter)	N_2		147

(continued)

Table 15 (continued)

Solvent	Concentration (mM)	Lasing wavelength (tuning) (nm)	Excitation	Output	Ref.
Hexafluoro-isopro-panol	1	690–743 (BF filter)	N_2		147
Ethanol + EG (1:19)			CW laser pumping		
Ethanol	0.15		Fl (60 J)	41 mJ	
DMSO		640–700 (grating)	N_2 (2 mJ, 8 ns, 5 Hz)	10 μJ	67
Methanol	0.025	660 (injection lock, ring cavity)	Fl	550 kW, 500 ns	149
Ethanol	2	660 (grating + prism)	N_2 (13 ns)	1.5 kW (3 ns)	
Acetone		598–650 (grating) (osc + amp)	YAG-SH (200 mJ)	E = 9%	98

Solvent	Conc.	Range (nm)	Pumping		Output
#M142 Resorufin					
Methanol		620–685 (grating) (osc + amp)	Laser pumping (pulse)	83	E = 10%
#M143 Resazurin					
Ethanol		610 (BB)	Laser pumping (pulse)	12	
Methanol or EG			Mode-locked HeNe (intracavity pumping)		
		662–724 (DFB)	Laser pumping (pulse)	148	
#M144 Oxazine 750					
DMSO + EG (1:4)	0.4 g/l	750–840 (BF filter)	Mode-locked Kr (647 nm, 0.3 W, 120–150 ps)	150	23 mWav. (18 ps) (syn-chronous pumping)
+ (SA:HDITC)		750–835 (BF filter)	0.4 W		12 mWav. (0.8 ps)

(continued)

121

Table 15 (continued)

Solvent	Concentration (mM)	Lasing wavelength (tuning) (nm)	Excitation	Output	Ref.
		770–785 (BF filter)	Mode-locked oxazine 1 laser (690 nm, 170 mW, 7 ps)	10–12 mW (1.1 ps)	142
		725–800	Cu (578 nm, 25 kW, 25 ns, 6 kHz)	E = 30%	50
EG + DMSO (85:15)	0.6	748–890	Kr (647 and 676 nm, 5 W)		26
EG + propylene carbonate		750–910 (BF filter) (ring cavity)	Mode-locked Kr (647 nm, 1W)	220 mW (3.2 ps) (synchronous pumping)	311
Propylene carbonate + EG	1.33	780–910 (BF filter)	Kr (647 and 676 nm, 4.7 W)	550 mW	312

Solvent		Wavelength	Laser		Ref.
#M145 Thionin					
Sulfuric acid		850 (BB)	Ruby		2
#M146 Methylene blue					
Sulfuric acid	$5 \times 10^{16} - 10^{17}$ cm^{-3}	835 (BB)	Ruby (0.5 J, 30–40 ns)	$E = 10\%$	6
Methanol	0.2	692 (BB)	Cresyl violet laser (64 nm, 11 MW, 10 Hz)	30 mWav.	36
#M147 Toluidine blue					
Sulfuric acid		848 (BB)	Ruby		2
#M148 Methylene green					
Sulfuric acid		823 (BB)	Ruby		2
#M149 Saphraine T					
Ethanol		610 (BB)	Glass-SH (8 MW)		76
Methanol		621–625 (BB)	Glass-SH		52

(continued)

Table 15 *(continued)*

^aStructures:

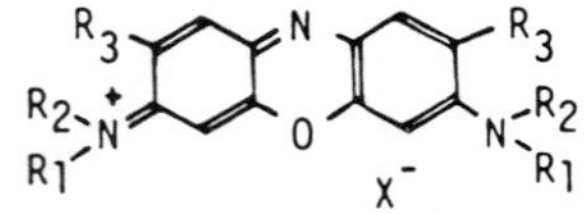

#M135 $R_1 = R_2 = R_3 = H$

#M136 $R_1 = R_2 = Et$, $R_3 = H$,
       $X = ClO_4$

#M137 $R_1 = Et$, $R_2 = H$,
       $R_3 = Me$, $X = ClO_4$

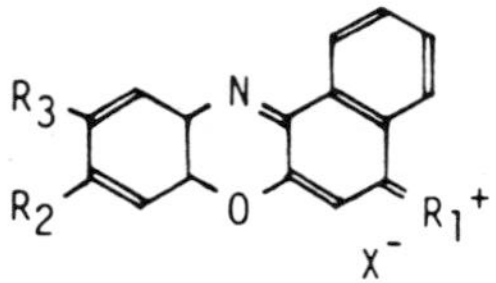

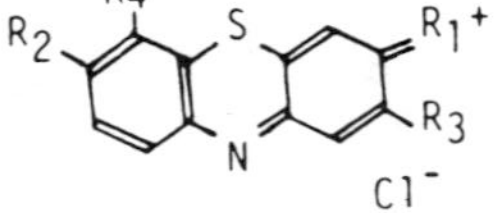

#M145 $R_1 = R_2 = NH_2$, $R_3 = R_4 = H$

#M146 $R_1 = R_2 = NMe_2$, $R_3 = R_4 = H$

#M147 $R_1 = NH_2$, $R_2 = NMe_2$, $R_3 = Me$, $R_4 = H$

#M148 $R_1 = R_2 = NMe_2$, $R_3 = H$, $R_4 = NO_2$

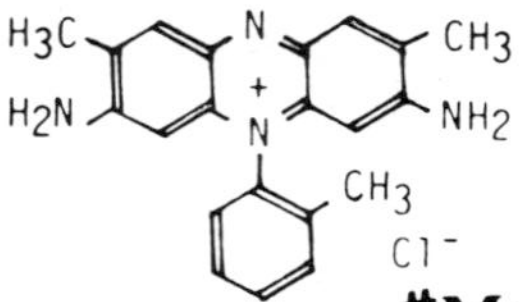

#M138 $R_1 = R_2 = NHEt$,
       $R_3 = Me$,
       $X = ClO_4$

#M139 $R_1 = NH_2$, $R_2 = N(Et)_2$,
       $R_3 = H$,
       $X = ClO_4$ or NO_3

#M140 $R_1 = R_2 = NH_2$, $R_3 = H$,
       $X = Cl$, ClO_4, CH_3CO_2,
       or NO_3

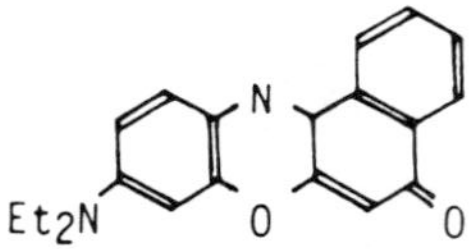

#M141

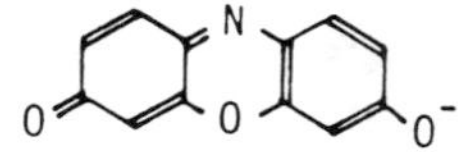

#M142

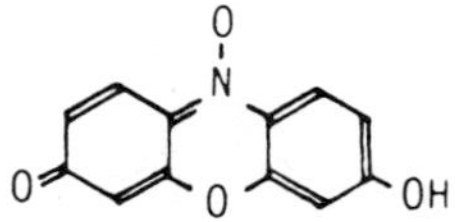

#M143

#M149

124

Table 16. Laser Characteristics of Chlorophylls[a]

Solvent	Concentration (mM)	Lasing wavelength (tuning) (nm)	Excitation	Output	Ref.
		#M150 Chlorophyll a			
Pyridine or ethanol	~2	677 and 681 (BB)	N_2 (1 MW)		151
		#M151 Chlorophyll b			
Pyridine	2	665 (BB)	N_2 (1 MW)		151
		#M152 Bacteriochlorophyll a			
Pyridine	1	800 (BB)	N_2 (1 MW)		151
		#M153 Pheophytin a			
Pyridine	1.2	680 and 725 (BB)	N_2 (1 MW)	(<1 ns for short cavity)	151

(continued)

Table 16 (continued)

Solvent	Concentration (mM)	Lasing wavelength (tuning) (nm)	Excitation	Output	Ref.
		#M154 Methyl pheophorbide a			
Pyridine		680 and 725 (BB)	N_2 (1 MW)		151

a Structures:

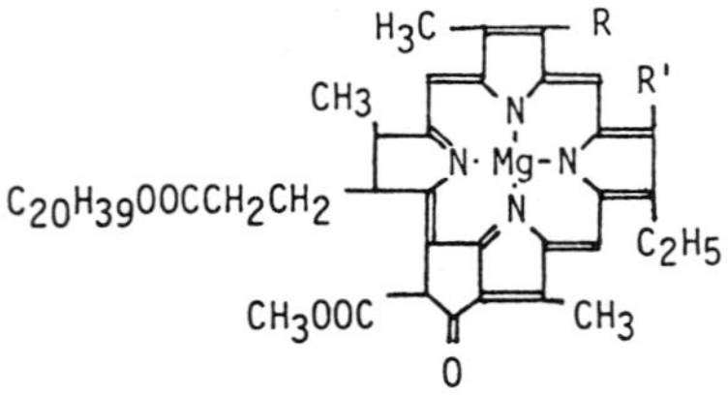

#M150 R = CHCH$_2$, R' = Me
#M151 R = CHCH$_2$, R' = CHO
#M152 R = COCH$_3$, R' = Me

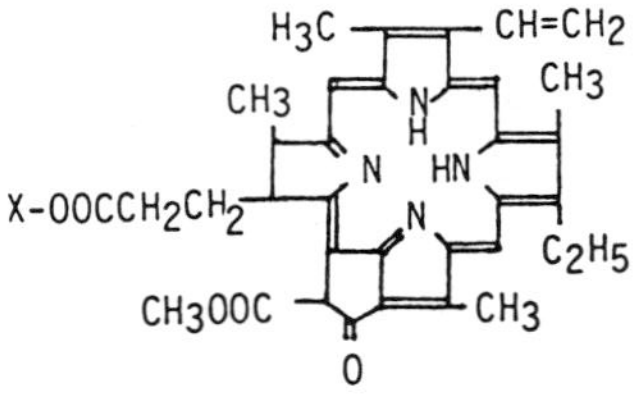

#M153 X = C$_{20}$H$_{39}$
#M154 X = Me

126

Table 17. Laser Characteristics of Other Dyes[a]

Solvent	Concentration (mM)	Lasing wavelength (tuning) (nm)	Excitation	Output	Ref.
		#M155 Amidopyrylium dye 140			
HFIP		720 (BB)	Fl		60
		#M156 Amidopyrylium dye 141			
HFIP		650 (BB)	Fl		60
		#M157 Carbopyronin 149			
Trifluoroethanol		650 (BB)	Fl		60
		#M158 Isoquinoline red			
Water		620 (BB)	Ruby-SH		2
		#M159 Rhodol			
Ethanol + DPB	0.15 + 2	564.5 (BB)	Fl (380 J, 38 μs)	80 mJ	81

(continued)

Table 17 (continued)

Solvent	Concentration (mM)	Lasing wavelength (tuning) (nm)	Excitation	Output	Ref.
		#M160 Violetrot			
Isoamyl alcohol		620 (BB)	Ruby or glass-SH		2
		610 (BB)	Fl		
		#M161 Pina (orthol)			
Ethanol		565 (BB)	Ruby-SH		2
		#M162 Rapid-filter gelt			
Isoamyl alcohol		620 (BB)	Ruby or glass-SH		2
		610 (BB)	Fl		
		#M163 Echtblau B			
Glycerin		753 (BB)	Ruby		2
		#M164 Rapid-filter grün			
Glycerin		795 (BB)	Ruby		2

128

#M165 Blatt grün

Solvent	Conc.	Wavelength	Laser/pump	Power	Ref.
Sulfuric acid		800 (BB)	Ruby		2
#M166 LD 690					
Methanol	0.28	660 (BB)	YAG–SH (10 Hz)		153
Ethanol + rhodamine 610	1.8 + 2.8	655–705	N_2		152
DMSO + ethanol (2:1) + rhodamine 610	2.5 + 2.8	660–716	N_2		
		680–730 (single axial mode, ring cavity)	Kr (647 and 676 nm, 6 W)	0.4 W	305
#M167 LD 700					
Alcohol		690 (BB)	Rhodamine 610 laser (YAG pump, 585 nm)		152
Ethanol	9.3 + 5	692–752	N_2		
+ rhodamine 640	1.5 + 4.4	698–758	N_2		

(continued)

129

Table 17 (*continued*)

Solvent	Concentration (mM)	Lasing wavelength (tuning) (nm)	Excitation	Output	Ref.
		690–780 (single axial mode, ring cavity)	Kr (647 and 676 nm, 4 W)	0.9 W	305
EG		700–840 (single axial mode, ring cavity)	Kr (all red lines, 6 W)	2 W	303
Benzyl alcohol + glycerin + DMSO + DCM (1:1)	1.2	700–805 (BF filter)	Kr (all blue-green lines, 4 W)	530 mW, E = 13%	304
Benzyl alcohol + EG + methanol + DCM	1.6	690–800 (BF filter)	Mode-locked Ar (514 nm, 1 Wav.)	70 mWav. (synchronous pumping)	313

[a]Structures:

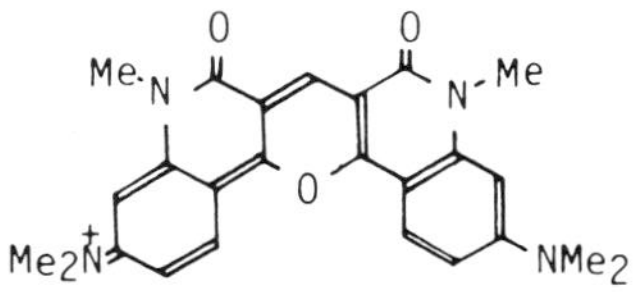

#M155

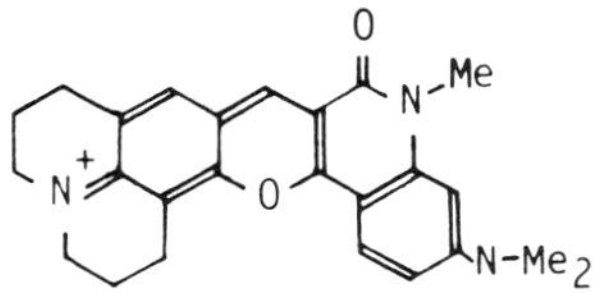

#M156

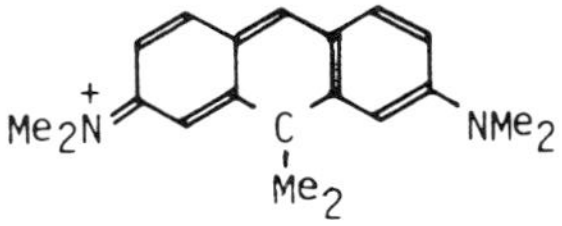

#M157

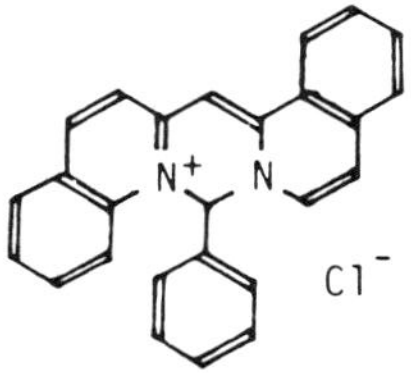

#M158

CHAPTER 5

Aromatic Compounds

In contrast to dyes, the lasing wavelengths of aromatic compounds are rather short. Anthracene and stilbene derivatives hold a majority in this class. From the practical point of view, however, oligophenylenes are important, because they are most efficient in the UV region. Some of the stilbene derivatives are also useful in the violet region.

I. Condensed Ring Compounds

A great many condensed-ring hydrocarbon compounds (see Fig. 7) and their derivatives show laser action (see Table 18). They are divided as follows:

1. Naphthalene (Fig. 7a)   #M168–#M170
2. Anthracene (Fig. 7b)   #M171–#M194
3. Fluorene (Fig. 7c)   #M195
4. Fluoranthene (Fig. 7d)   #M196
5. Tetracene (Fig. 7e)   #M197
6. Pyrene (Fig. 7f)   #M198–#M201
7. Perylene (Fig. 7g)   #M202–#M204
8. Coronene (Fig. 7h)   #M205

133

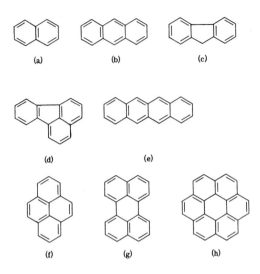

(a)   (b)   (c)

(d)   (e)

(f)   (g)   (h)

Fig. 7. Structures of condensed ring compounds: (a) naphthalene, (b) anthracene, (c) fluorene, (d) fluoranthene, (e) tetracene, (f) pylene, (g) perylene, and (h) coronene.

Most of these compounds have a high fluorescence quantum yield. However, their lasing efficiencies are poor in general. This may be caused by the remarkable triplet-state absorption. Even for short-pulse (~10 ns) excitation, remarkable quenching is observed in the trailing portion of the lasing pulse. Therefore, lasing is difficult for slow-rising excitation like flashlamps. Various derivatives of anthracene are well known as efficient fluorescence materials. Aristov *et al.* have investigated these anthracene derivatives and reported that deoxygenation of the solvent improves the lasing efficiency (160). The lasing wavelengths are in violet or blue, and become longer as the number of benzene rings increases. Some of the sulfonic salts of pyrene (#M198–#M200) are pumpable by flashlamps.

II. Oligophenylenes

p-Oligophenylenes are generally composed of benzene rings joined together in the para position as shown in Fig. 8. Laser action is reported for the following three classes of compounds (see Table 19):

1. p-Terphenyl (n = 3) (Fig. 8a)   #M206–#M208
2. p-Quaterphenyl (n = 4) (Fig. 8b)   #M209–#M212
3. p-Qinquiephenyl (n = 5) (Fig. 8c)   #M213

No laser action takes place for biphenyl (n = 2), whose quantum yield is small. Its resonance wavelengths shift toward longer wavelengths as the number of benzene rings increases (139).

These are very important materials in the UV region shorter than 400 nm. p-Terphenyl (#M206) is a valuable efficient compound in UV. BM-terphenyl (#M208) is known as the lasing compound at the shortest wavelengths. The short wavelength limit is 308.5 nm (243,302). The shortest limit in CW operation is 362 nm, which is attained with polyphenyl 1 (#M212), a derivative of p-quaterphenyl (242). KrF and XeCl excimer lasers, and FHG of Nd:YAG laser are their good pumping sources. Flashlamp pumping is possible, but a first risetime (<100 ns) is required (137,179).

Generally, aromatic solvents are utilized for these compounds. The solubility is drastically reduced as n increases. In the case of UV pumping, one must take care of the absorption by the solvent. Cyclohexane is a recommended solvent because it is transparent down to 220 nm.

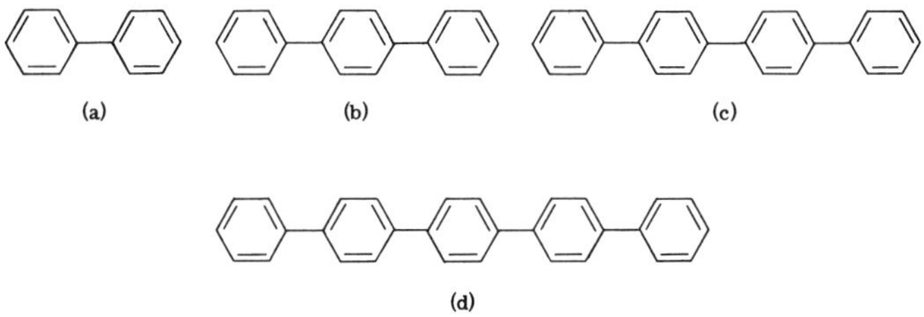

(a)   (b)   (c)

(d)

Fig. 8. Structures of oligophenylenes: (a) biphenyl, (b) p-terphenyl, (c) p-quaterphenyl, and (d) p-quinquiephenyl.

Wood *et al.* (187) and Abakumov *et al.* (240) have discussed the possibility of the dye laser action at wavelengths shorter than 300 nm.

III. Conjugated Diene Compounds

These are derivatives of uncyclic unsaturated hydrocarbons such as ethylene and butadiene (see Tables 20 and 21). Most of them are terminated by phenyl radicals. Derivatives of stilbene (Fig. 9a) and distryl benzene (bistilbene, Fig. 9b) are important in this class. The tunable ranges of these stilbene compounds are 400–500 nm. They are chemically stable, but their laser performances are inferior to those of coumarins. Therefore, they are useful at the wavelengths shorter than 430 nm at which laser action of coumarin is difficult.

Stilbene 3 (#M260), a sulfonated bistilbene, shows efficient CW laser action with a tunable range from 403 to 493 nm (199). Some of the stilbene compounds are known as useful fluorescent whitening agents. Majewski and Krasinski have reported laser action in many fluorescent whitening agents by the excitation of an N_2 laser (198).

IV. Miscellaneous Aromatic Compounds

Table 22 lists miscellaneous compounds including benzene derivatives (#M271 and #M272).

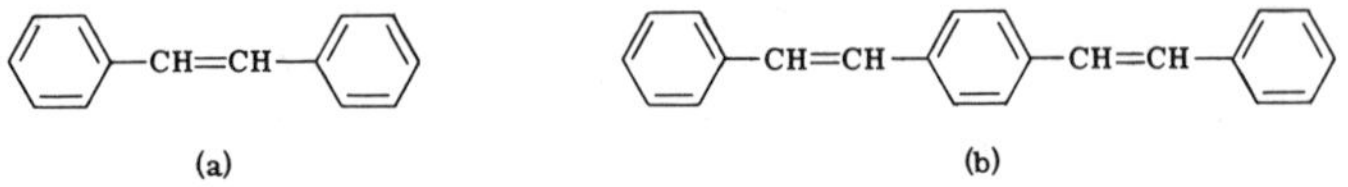

(a)   (b)

Fig. 9. Structures of (a) stilbene and (b) distrylbenzene (bistilbene).

Table 18. Laser Characteristics of Condensed Ring Compounds[a,b]

Solvent	Concentration (mM)	Lasing wavelength (tuning) (nm)	Excitation	Output	Ref.
#M168 (3-Carboxy-2-hydroxy-1-naphthyl)methyleneiminodiacetic acid					
Water + Sr^{2+}, Ca^{2+}, Ba^{2+} (pH 12.4–12.7)	28–43	490 (BB)	N$_2$ (25 kW, 10 ns)		154
#M169 2-Naphthole-6,8-disulfonic acid dipotassium salt					
Water	1	475 (BB)	N$_2$ (1 MW, 2.5 ns)		155
#M170 Amino G acid; 7-amino-1,3-naphthalenedisulfonic acid					
Water	8	459 (BB)	Fl (9 J, 80 ns, RT)	Thr = 5.1 J	1
#M171 Anthracene					
Fluorene (crystal)	2	408 (BB)	N$_2$ (1 kW, 4 ns)	10 W$_{peak}$ (<3 ns)	156

(continued)

Table 18 *(continued)*

Solvent	Concentration (mM)	Lasing wavelength (tuning) (nm)	Excitation	Output	Ref.
2,3-Dimethyl-naphthalene (crystal)	1	408-410 (BB)	N_2 (2 kW, 3-4 ns)	100 W (3 ns)	157
#M172 9-Chloroanthracene					
Methanol + ethanol (1:4)	10	415.5-415.8 (BB, 154-195 K)	N_2 (100 kW, 10 ns, 100 Hz)	(3.5 ns)	158
#M173 9-Phenylanthracene					
Methanol + ethanol (1:4)	10	417.3-417.5 (BB, 160-192 K)	N_2 (100 kW, 10 ns, 100 Hz)	(4.3 ns)	158
#M174 9-Methylanthracene					
Methanol + ethanol (1:4)	10	413.8-414.1 (BB, 156-202 K)	N_2 (100 kW, 10 ns, 100 Hz)	(4.5 ns)	158

#M175 9,10-Diphenylanthracene

Solvent		Wavelength	Laser		Ref.
Cyclo-hexane	10	432.6 (BB)	Ruby-SH (1 MW)		159
		435-450 (grating)	N_2 (120 kW, 10 ns, 100 Hz)	E = 8% (2 ns)	130
Methanol + ethanol (1:4)	5	429.3-430.2 (BB, 164-192 K)	N_2 (100 kW, 10 ns, 100 Hz)	(4 ns)	158
Methyl-cyclo-hexane + toluene (2:1)		431.7-436.6 (BB, 149-295 K)		(2.5 ns)	
Toluene (deoxy-genated)	5	435 (BB)	Ruby-SH (0.03 J, 20 ns)		160

#M176 2-Chloro-9,10-diphenylanthracene

Solvent		Wavelength	Laser	Ref.
Toluene (deoxy-genated)	5	439 (BB)	Ruby-SH (0.03 J, 20 ns)	160

(continued)

Table 18 *(continued)*

Solvent	Concentration (mM)	Lasing wavelength (tuning) (nm)	Excitation	Output	Ref.
		#M177 2-(α-Hydroxyethyl)-9,10-diphenylanthracene			
Toluene (deoxy- genated	5	439 (BB)	Ruby–SH (0.03 J, 20 ns)		160
		#M178 9,10-Di-(p-bromophenyl)anthracene			
Toluene (deoxy- genated	5	439 (BB)	Ruby–SH (0.03 J, 20 ns)		160
		#M179 9,10-Di-(o-tolyl)anthracene			
Toluene	2	427 (BB)	Ruby–SH (0.03 J, 20 ns)		160
		#M180 9,10-Di-(m-tolyl)anthracene			
Toluene (deoxy- genated)	5	435 (BB)	Ruby–SH (0.03 J, 20 ns)		160

#M181 9,10-Di-(p-tolyl)anthracene

Toluene (deoxygenated)	5	439 (BB)	Ruby-SH (0.03 J, 20 ns)		160

#M182 9,10-Dichloroanthracene

Toluene (deoxygenated)	5	435 (BB)	Ruby-SH (0.03 J, 20 ns)		160
Isoamyl acetate	8.7	429–435 (BB)	N_2 (100 kW, 5 ns)	3 kW	161

#M183 9,10-Dimethylanthracene

Methyl-cyclohexane + toluene (2:1)	10	432–432.7 (BB, 202–230 K)	N_2 (100 kW, 10 ns, 100 Hz)	(4.2 ns)	158
Toluene (deoxygenated)	5	435 (BB)	Ruby-SH (0.03 J, 20 ns)		160

(continued)

Table 18 *(continued)*

Solvent	Concentration (mM)	Lasing wavelength (tuning) (nm)	Excitation	Output	Ref.
#M184 9,10-Diethylanthracene					
Toluene (deoxy-genated)	5	433 (BB)	Ruby-SH (0.03 J, 20 ns)		160
#M185 9,10-Di-(*n*-propyl)anthracene					
Toluene (deoxy-genated)	5	433 (BB)	Ruby-SH (0.03 J, 20 ns)		160
#M186 9-*n*-Propyl-10-(1-propenyl)anthracene					
Toluene (deoxy-genated)	5	457 (BB)	Ruby-SH (0.03 J, 20 ns)		160
#M187 9,10-Diallylanthracene					
Toluene	5	431 (BB)	Ruby-SH (0.03 J, 20 ns)		160

142

#M188 9,10-Di-(n-butyl)anthracene					
Toluene (deoxygenated)	5	435 (BB)	Ruby-SH (0.03 J, 20 ns)		160
Toluene	5	463 (BB)			160
#M189 9,10-Di-(p-anisyl)anthracene					
Toluene (deoxygenated)	5	446 (BB)	Ruby-SH (0.03 J, 20 ns)		160
#M190 9,10-Di-(o-anisyl)anthracene					
Toluene	2	446 (BB)	Ruby-SH (0.03 J, 20 ns)		160
#M191 2-Chloro-9,10-di-(n-propyl)anthracene					
Toluene (deoxygenated)	5	439 (BB)	Ruby-SH (0.03 J, 20 ns)		160
#M192 10-Phenyl-9-acetoxyanthracene					
Dioxane	50	414 and 427.5 (BB)	N_2 (350 kW, 10 ns)	(ASE)	162

(continued)

Table 18 (continued)

Solvent	Concentration (mM)	Lasing wavelength (tuning) (nm)	Excitation	Output	Ref.
		#M193 10-(4-Acetoxyphenyl)-9-acetoxyanthracene			
Dioxane	50	417.7 and 428.3 (BB)	N_2 (350 kW, 10 ns)	(ASE)	162
		#M194 10-(4-Methylphenyl)-9-acetoxyanthracene			
Dioxane	50	431 (BB)	N_2 (350 kW, 10 ns)	(ASE)	162
		#M195 2-Amino-7-nitrofluorene			
Dichloro-benzene	4-5	540-585 (BB, concentration)	Ruby-SH (300 MW, 20 ns, fundamental)		163
		#M196 3-Aminofluoranthene			
Ethanol (deoxy-genated)	60 mg/1	548-580	Fl (100 J, 800 ns, RT)		74

#M197 Tetracene

p-Terphenyl (crystal)	1	530 (BB)	N$_2$ (2 kW, 3–4 ns)		157
Dibenzyl (crystal)	10^{16} cm^{-3}	494 and 521 (BB) 4.2 K	Nd–THG (2 MW, 30 ns)	E = 25%	207

#M198 8-Hydroxypylene-1,3,6-trisulfonic acid (sodium salt); pyrene 1

Water (base)		550 (BB)	Fl		60
Water (base)		539 (BB)	Fl (30 J)	Thr = 9 J	165

#M199 3-Ethylaminopyrene-5,8,10-trisulfonic acid (sodium salt)

Water	2.5	441 (BB)	Ruby-SH (200 kW)		24
Water		547–554 (BB)	Ruby-SH, Fl		52

#M200 8-Acetamidopyrene-1,3,6-trisulfonic acid (sodium salt)

Water or methanol	1	Green-yellow	Fl (300 ns, RT)		75
Water		441–453 (BB)	Ruby-SH, Fl		52

(continued)

Table 18 *(continued)*

Solvent	Concentration (mM)	Lasing wavelength (tuning) (nm)	Excitation	Output	Ref.
Water (base)		566-574 (BB)			
		#M201 1,3,6,8-Tetraphenylpyrene			
Benzene	2.5	422-430 (BB)	Ruby-SH (5 MW, 20 ns)	0.8 MW	164
		#M202 Perylene			
DMF	1.3	471 (BB)	N_2 (200 kW, 3 ns, 10 Hz)	1.5 kW	71
Cyclo-hexane	0.17	465.6 (BB)	N_2 (200 kW, 3 ns, 10 Hz)	1.4 kW	
Benzene	0.1-0.05	473 (BB)	Ruby-SH (4 MW, 30 ns)	0.3 MW	166
DMF	0.8	476 (BB)	Ruby-SH (8 MW, 8 ns)	0.4 MW	73
Benzene	1.6 g/l	473 (BB)	N_2 (50 kW, 7 ns)	Thr = 19.5 kV (ASE)	167

+ PPO	1.6 + 2 g/l	473 (BB)		Thr = 15.5 kV	
+ bis-MSB	0.05 + 3.6 g/l	420, 447, and 473 (BB)		Thr = 16.8-18.5 kV	155

#M203 1,6,7,12-Tetracarboxy perylene

Water + NaOH	1	517 (BB)	N_2 (1 MW, 2.5 ns)		

#M204 1,7-Bis(n-butoxycarbonyl)perylene

PMMA	10^{17} cm^{-3}	509 (BB)	Glass-Th (0.04 J, 40 ns)		168
	10^{18} cm^{-3}	514 (BB)			

#M205 Coronene

Methyl-cyclo-hexane + iso-pentane	0.1	443.9 (BB, 100 K)	Fl (625 J, 0.5-5 μs)	Thr = 50 J	169

[a] Recently 8 new acetoxy-phenyl anthracene derivatives have been reported (296).

(continued)

Table 18 (continued)

b Structures:

#M168

#M169 R=KSO$_3$, R'=OH
#M170 R=HSO$_3$, R'=NH$_2$

#M171— #M194

#M195

#M196

#M197

#M198 R=SO$_3$Na, R'=OH
#M199 R=SO$_3$Na, R'=NHEt
#M200 R=SO$_3$Na, R'=NHAc
#M201 R=R'=Ph

#M202 R=R'=H
#M203 R=R'=COOH
#M204 R=CO$_2$C$_4$H$_9$, R'=H

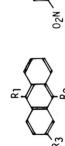

#M205

Dye no.	R_1	R_2	R_3		Dye no.	R_1	R_2	R_3
#M171	H	H	H		#M183	Me	Me	H
#M172	Cl	H	H		#M184	Et	Et	H
#M173	Ph	H	H		#M185	n-Pr	n-Pr	H
#M174	Me	H	H		#M186	n-Pr	CHCHCH$_3$	H
#M175	Ph	Ph	H		#M187	Allyl	Allyl	H
#M176	Ph	Ph	Cl		#M188	n-Bu	n-Bu	H
#M177	Ph	Ph	CHOHCH$_3$		#M189	p-As	p-As	H
#M178	p-BrPh	p-BrPh	H		#M190	o-As	o-As	H
#M179	o-Tl	o-Tl	H		#M191	n-Pr	n-Pr	Cl
#M180	m-Tl	m-Tl	H		#M192	Ph	OAc	H
#M181	p-Tl	p-Tl	H		#M193	p-OAc-Ph	OAc	H
#M182	Cl	Cl	H		#M194	p-Tl	OAc	H

149

Table 19. Laser Characteristics of Oligophenylenes[a]

#M206 p-Terpheny; PTP; U.V. 1

Solvent	Concentration (mM)	Lasing wavelength (tuning) (nm)	Excitation	Output	Ref.
Cyclohexane	1.3	341 (BB)	Glass-FH (0.5-0.6 MW)	E = 1.3%	177
Cyclohexane	1	330-360 (grating)	Glass-FH	Thr = 100 kW	178
DMF	0.8	341 (BB)	Fl (20 J, 50 ns, RT)	40 kW (ASE), Thr = 6.6 J, Thr = 4.2 J	137
Dioxane	0.2-0.4	342.5-355.5 (BB, concentration)			
Cyclohexane	9	340 (BB)	CO_2-laser-produced plasma (5.6 J)	0.1 mJ (25 ns)	115
Cyclohexane	2	342.6 (BB)	Fl (81.5 J, 80 ns, RT)	25.2 mJ, 0.42 MW	179
Dioxane	10	335-346 (grating)	KrF (1 mJ, 25 ns)	25 μJ, 3 kW	180

Solvent	Conc.	Tuning	Laser	Output	Ref.
Cyclohexane	1–5	323–364 (grating)	KrF (6 mJ, 5 ns, 100 Hz)	E = 28%	181
Cyclohexane	0.08	321.8–365.3 (grating)	KrF (8 MW, 15 ns)	1 MW, 11 mJ, E = 10%	59
Cyclohexane	2	340.3 (BB)	XeCl (60 mJ, 35 ns)	E = 20.7%	95
Cyclohexane	5	334–362	KrF	80 kW, E = 30%	182
			XeBr	E = 20%	
		340 (BB)	Mode-locked glass–FH (4 mJ, 7 ps, single pulse)	75 µJ, E = 5% (ps pulse)	93
Cyclohexane	2	333–348 (grating) (osc + amp)	YAG–FH (5 mJ, 5 ns, 10 Hz)	E = 6%	183
Cyclohexane	4	334–347 (grating) (osc + amp)	KrF, XeCl (150–250 mJ, 10–20 ns)	E = 14%	26
Dioxane		343 (BB)	XeCl (3.5 J)	1 J, E = 29%	306

(continued)

Table 19 (continued)

Solvent	Concentration (mM)	Lasing wavelength (tuning) (nm)	Excitation	Output	Ref.
	#M207	4,4'-N,N,N',N'-Tetraethylamino-p-terphenyl			
DMF		417–427 (BB)	Fl (200 ns, RT)	Thr = 26 J	184
	#M208	2,2"-Dimethyl-p-terphenyl; BM-terphenyl			
Cyclohexane	0.96	311.2–360 (grating)	KrF (70 mJ, 14 ns)	9 mJ	243
Cyclohexane	0.9	311–350 (grating) (osc + amp)	KrF (250 mJ, 10–20 ns)	E = 8%	26
EPA (77 K)	0.7	308.5– (grating)	KrF		302
		#M209 p-Quaterphenyl			
Toluene		362–390 (grating)	N$_2$ (100 kW, 10 ns)		185
DMF	7	374 (BB)	Fl (20 J, 50 ns, RT)	Thr = 6 J	137

Solvent	Conc.	Wavelength	Laser (pump conditions)	Output	Ref.
DMF	Satur.	370 (BB)	N_2 (530 kW, 3.5 ns)	E = 11%	139
DMF	0.075	375 (BB)	Fl (100 J, 150 ns, RT)	12 mJ	186
Cyclohexane	1	365 (BB)	CO_2-laser-produced plasma (10 J)	0.2 mJ	187
Vapor, SF_6 (10 atm)	280°C	350 (BB)	Nd-FH (5-20 mJ, 15 ns)	E = 1%	188

#M210 4,4'''-Bisbutyloctyloxy-*p*-quaterphenyl; BBQ; BBOQ; pilot 386; U.V. 3; BiBuQ

Solvent	Conc.	Wavelength	Laser (pump conditions)	Output	Ref.
Buthanol		381–389 (BB)	Fl (200 ns, RT)	Thr = 13 J	184
Hexane emulsified in glycerin + water	1	(BB)	N_2 (50 kW)		191
Dioxane		380.3 (grating + prism)	KrF (20 mJ, 10 ns, 7 Hz)	30 kW	189
Dioxane or cyclohexane	2.6	386 (BB)	KrF (160 mJ, 0.2 Wav.)	11 mJ (10–12 ns)	190
			XeCl (60 mJ, 35 ns)	E = 25.1%	
Dioxane	0.5	383.4 (BB)	N_2 (3.5 mJ, 15 ns)	E = 18.8%	95

(continued)

153

Table 19 *(continued)*

Solvent	Concentration (mM)	Lasing wavelength (tuning) (nm)	Excitation	Output	Ref.
Ethanol + toluene (1:1)	2	380–410 (etalon)	Mode-locked YAG–TH (1 GW, 30 ps/pulse)	A few MW (25 ps) (synchronous pumping)	192
Cyclohexane	2.5	373–391 (grating) (osc + amp)	YAG–FH (5 mJ, 5 ns, 10 Hz)	E = 3.8%	183
Cyclohexane		360–395 (grating) (osc + amp)	XeCl (55 mJ, 10 Hz)	9 mJ, E = 16%	242
Toluene + ethanol (1:1)	2.5	373–399 (grating) (osc + amp)	N$_2$ (1 MW, 10 ns, 50 Hz)	0.85 mJ	97
Cyclohexane	0.36	359–405 (grating) (osc + amp)	XeCl (150 mJ, 10–20 ns)	E = 17%	26

| DMF | 0.08 | 370–410 (grating) | F1 (150 ns, RT, 1 Hz) | | 87 |

#M211 3,3',2'',3'''-Tetramethyl-p-quaterphenyl; TMQ

| Cyclohexane | 2 | 338–361 (grating) (osc + amp) | YAG-FH (5 mJ, 5 ns, 10 Hz) | E = 1.2% | 183 |
| Cyclohexane | 2 | 338–360 (grating) (osc + amp) | KrF or XeCl (150–250 mJ, 10–20 ns) | E = 6% | 26 |

#M212 Polyphenyl 1

EG	0.2–0.6	360–410 (grating) (osc + amp)	XeCl (55 mJ, 10 Hz)	10.2 mJ, E = 18.5%	242
EG	2.5	362–412 (BF filter)	Ar (UV all lines, 3.3 W)	80 mW, Thr = 1 W	242
EG	0.56	360–408 (grating) (osc + amp)	XeCl (150 mJ, 10–20 ns)	E = 18%	26
EG	2.5	360–415 (grating) (osc + amp)	N_2 (1.5 MW, 4 ns)	E = 14%	26

(continued)

Table 19 (continued)

Solvent	Concentration (mM)	Lasing wavelength (tuning) (nm)	Excitation	Output	Ref.
		#M213 p-Quinquephenyl			
Dioxane	Satur.	420 (BB)	N_2 (530 kW, 3.5 ns)	E = 15.5%	139
		#M214 p-Phenylene-4,4'-bistetraphenylimidazole-2-diium dichloride			
Ethanol	Satur.	426 (BB)	N_2 (1 MW, 2.5 ns)		155
		#M215 p-Terphenylene-4,4''-bis(tetraphenylimidazole-2-diium)dichloride			
Ethanol	Satur.	415 (BB)	N_2 (1 MW, 2.5 ns)		155

^{a}Structures:

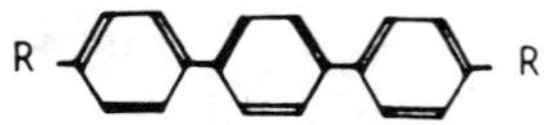

#M206 R = H
#M207 R = NEt$_2$

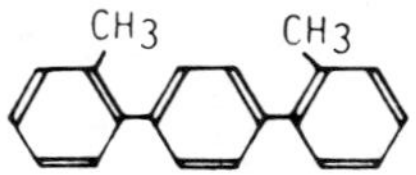

#M208

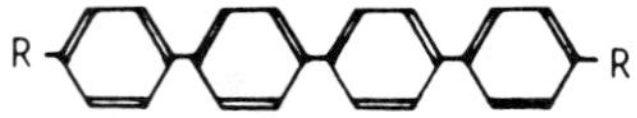

#M209 R = H
#M210 R = -O-CH$_2$-CH-C$_6$H$_{13}$
                          |
                        C$_4$H$_9$

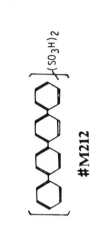

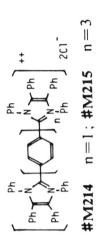

$(SO_3H)_2$

#M212

#M211

#M213

$2Cl^-$

#M214 n = 1 ; **#M215** n = 3

Table 20. Laser Characteristics of Conjugated Diene Compounds[a]

Solvent	Concentration (mM)	Lasing wavelength (tuning) (nm)	Excitation	Output	Ref.
#M216 4-Phenylstilbene; PBE					
Dioxane	2	380 (BB)	N_2 (530 kW, 3.5 ns)	E = 0.8%	139
Naphthalene (crystal)	2×10^{17} cm^{-3}	376 (BB) 4.2 K	Nd-THG (2 MW, 30 ns)		207
#M217 4,4'-Diphenylstilbene; 1,2-di-4-biphenylylethylene; DPS; BBE					
Toluene		408 (BB)	Glass-TH (1 MW)		76
Benzene	1	408.5 (BB)	Ruby-SH (0.8 MW, 12 ns)		193
Benzene	Satur. ×0.66	409 (BB)	Fl (20 J, 50 ns, RT)	Thr = 3.8 J	137
Benzene		400–420 (grating)	N_2 (120 kW, 10 ns, 100 Hz)	E = 23% (8 ns)	130
Xylene	Satur.	404.6–411.7 (grating)	N_2 (100 kW)		194

Benzene	0.25	406 (BB)	Fl (100 J, 150 ns, RT)	10 mJ	186
		405 (BB)	Mode-locked glass–TH (1–3 mJ, 6 ps, single pulse)	0.1 mJ, E = 5% (ps pulse)	93
Dioxane	<1.2	401–404 (BF filter)	Xe (364 nm, 5 kW, 200 ns, 10 Hz)	500 W, E = 10% (120 ns)	195
Dioxane	Satur.	405.5 (BB)	XeCl (60 mJ, 35 ns)	E = 27.3%	95
Dioxane	Satur.	396–416 (grating) (osc + amp)	N_2 (1 MW, 10 ns, 50 Hz)	0.8 mJ	97
Dioxane	0.7	393–419 (grating) (osc + amp)	XeCl (150 mJ, 10–20 ns)	E = 13%	26
Biphenyl (crystal)		418 (BB) 4.2 K	Nd–THG (2 MW, 30 ns)		207
#M218 Stilbene 1; sulphonated diphenylstilbene					
EG	1	390.4–448.5 (BF filter)	Kr (UV all lines, 3.7 W)	440 mW, E = 12%	196

(continued)

159

Table 20 (continued)

Solvent	Concentration (mM)	Lasing wavelength (tuning) (nm)	Excitation	Output	Ref.
EG	0.67 g/liter	395–435 (BF filter)	Ar or Kr (UV all lines, 3 W)	300 mW, E = 12%	86
		405–428 (single axial mode)		58 mW	
EG	1	398–435 (grating) (osc + amp)	XeCl (150 mJ, 10–20 ns)	E = 16%	26
EG	0.6	390–450 (grating) (osc + amp)	N_2 (1.5 MW, 4 ns)	E = 17%	
EG + BZ		405–428 (ring cavity, single axial mode)	Ar (UV all lines, 3 W)	150 mW	303

#M219 1-(4-Biphenyl)-2-(1-naphthyl)ethylene; α NBE

Solvent	Concentration (mM)	Lasing wavelength (tuning) (nm)	Excitation	Output	Ref.
Cyclohexane	0.8	410.8 (BB)	Ruby (5 MW, 20 ns)	0.3 MW	164
Benzene		416.6 (BB)			

#M220 1,2-Di(1-naphthyl)ethylene; α NNE

Toluene		426 (BB)	Glass-TH (1 MW)		76

#M221 1,2-Di(2-naphthyl)ethylene; β NNE

Naphthalene (crystal)	10^{18} cm^{-3}	397 (BB) 4.2 K	Nd-THG (2 MW, 30 ns)	E = 25%	207

#M222 1-(4-Biphenyl)-2-(2-naphthyl)ethylene; β NBE

Naphthalene (crystal)	10^{18} cm^{-3}	397 (BB) 4.2 K	Nd-THG (2 MW, 30 ns)	Thr = 0.01 J/cm^2	207

#M223 1-(1-Naphthyl)-2-(2-naphthyl)ethylene

Naphthalene (crystal)		397 (BB) 4.2 K	Nd-THG (2 MW, 30 ns)		207

#M224 1-(2-Naphthyl)-2-phenylethylene

Naphthalene (crystal)	10^{18} cm^{-3}	385 (BB) 4.2 K	Nd-THG (2 MW, 30 ns)	Thr = 0.01 J/cm^2	207

#M225 4,4'-Bis(4-phenyl-2H-triazol-2-yl)-2,2'-stilbenedisulfonic acid dipotssium salt; triazinyl stilbene No. 10

Water + NP-10	1.5	420-454 (grating)	N$_2$ (100 kW, 7 ns, 75 Hz)	E = 3.6%	197

(continued)

Table 20 *(continued)*

Solvent	Concentration (mM)	Lasing wavelength (tuning) (nm)	Excitation	Output	Ref.
Methanol	1.5	414-437.5 (grating)		E = 3.6%	
		#M226 Tinopal PCRP; FBA 70			
Benzene	1	430 (BB)	N_2 (1 MW, 2.5 ns)		155
Dioxane		414-453 (prism)	N_2 (200 kW, 6 ns, 30 Hz)		198
		#M227 Tinopal RBS; FBA 46			
Methanol + dioxane (1:9)		414-472 (prism)	N_2 (200 kW, 6 ns, 30 Hz)		198
		#M228 Tinopal GS; FBA 47			
Methanol		422-476 (prism)	N_2 (200 kW, 6 ns, 30 Hz)		198

Compound	Solvent		Laser		Ref.
#M229 Blankophor R; FBA 30	Methanol	396–447 (prism)	N$_2$ (200 kW, 6 ns, 30 Hz)		198
#M230 Delft weiss BSW; FBA 81	Methanol	411–464 (prism)	N$_2$ (200 kW, 6 ns, 30 Hz)		198
#M231 Tinopal BV; FBA 1	Methanol	405–459 (prism)	N$_2$ (200 kW, 6 ns, 30 Hz)		198
#M232 Leukophor B; FBA 32	Methanol	410–465 (prism)	N$_2$ (200 kW, 6 ns, 30 Hz)		198
#M233 Uvitex CF; FBA 134; weisstoner BV; FBA 111	Methanol	410–462 (prism)	N$_2$ (200 kW, 6 ns, 30 Hz)		198
#M234 4,4'-Bis[(4-anilino-6-methoxy-1,3,5-triazin-2-yl)amino]-2,2'-stilbenedisulfonic acid; triazinyl stilbene No. 1	Water + NP10	1.5	417.5–442.5 (grating)	N$_2$ (100 kW, 7 ns, 75 Hz)	E = 2.2%	197

(continued)

163

Table 20 (continued)

Solvent	Concentration (mM)	Lasing wavelength (tuning) (nm)	Excitation	Output	Ref.
#M235 4,4'-Bis[[4-anilino-6-(2-hydroxyethylamino)-1,3,5-triazin-2-yl]amino]-2,2'-stilbenedisulfonic acid; triazinyl stilbene No. 2					
Water + NP-10	1.5	420-438 (grating)	N_2 (100 kW, 7 ns, 75 Hz)	E = 2.5%	197
#M236 4,4'-Bis[[6-bis(2-hydroxypropyl)amino-4-(x-sulfoanilino)-1,3,5-triazin-2-yl]amino]-2,2'-stilbenedisulfonic acid; tryazinyl stilbene No. 3					
Water + NP-10	1.5	420-447 (grating)	N_2 (100 kW, 7 ns, 75 Hz)	E = 2.8%	197
#M237 4,4'-Bis[[6-bis(2-hydroxyethyl)amino-4-(x-sulfoanilino)-1,3,5-triazin-2-yl]amino]-2,2'-stilbenedisulfonic acid; tryazinyl stilbene No. 4					
Water + NP-10	1.6	425-459 (grating)	N_2 (100 kW, 7 ns, 75 Hz)	E = 3.2%	197

Solvent	Conc.	Wavelength range	Pump	Efficiency	Ref.
Methanol	1.6	417.5-461 (grating)		E = 3.2%	199
EG + methanol (9:1)	2	411-481 (BF filter)	Ar (UV all lines, 3.5 W)	350 mW	199

#M238 4,4'-Bis[[6-(2-hydroxyethyl)methylamino-4-(x-sulfoanilino)-1,3,5-triazin-2-yl]amino]-2,2'-stilbenedisulfonic acid; tryazinyl stilbene No. 5

Solvent	Conc.	Wavelength range	Pump	Efficiency	Ref.
Water + NP-10	1.5	420-445 (grating)	N_2 (100 kW, 7 ns, 75 Hz)	E = 2.6%	197

#M239 4,4'-Bis[[4-(x,y-disulfoanilino)-6-morpholino-1,3,5-triazin-2-yl]amino]-2,2'-stilbenedisulfonic acid; tryazinyl stilbene No. 6

Solvent	Conc.	Wavelength range	Pump	Efficiency	Ref.
Water + NP-10	1.5	418-448 (grating)	N_2 (100 kW, 7 ns, 75 Hz)	E = 2.95%	197

#M240 4,4'-Bis[[4-(x,y-disulfoanilino)-6-(2-hydroxyethyl)methylamino-1,3,5-triazin-2-yl]amino]-2,2'-stilbenedisulfonic acid; tryazinyl stilbene No. 7

Solvent	Conc.	Wavelength range	Pump	Efficiency	Ref.
Water + NP-10	1.5	418-449 (grating)	N_2 (100 kW, 7 ns, 75 Hz)	E = 2.95%	197

(continued)

Table 20 *(continued)*

Solvent	Concentration (mM)	Lasing wavelength (tuning) (nm)	Excitation	Output	Ref.
#M241 4,4'-Bis[[4-(x,y-disulfoanilino)-6-ethylamino-1,3,5-triazin-2-yl]amino]-2,2'-stilbenedisulfonic acid; tryazinyl stilbene No. 8					
Water + NP-10	1.5	419-447.5 (grating)	N$_2$ (100 kW, 7 ns, 75 Hz)	E = 3.2%	197
#M242 1,4-Distyryl benzene					
Toluene		415 (BB)	Glass-TH (1 MW)		76
Toluene	1.6	411 and 417 (BB)	Glass-TH (8 MW)	E = 7.5%	177
Toluene	~1	412-435 (grating)	N$_2$ (600 kW, 5 ns, 5-50 Hz)	45 kW	200
#M243 1,4-Bis(2-methylstyryl)benzene; bis MSB					
Ethanol	0.1	419 (BB)	Ruby-SH (0.8 MW, 12 ns)		193

Toluene	0.4	424 (BB)	Fl (90 J, 100 ns, RT)	12 kW, Thr = 44 J	138
Dioxane	3.5	423 (BB, short cavity)	Mode-locked YAG-TH (1 mJ, 11 ps, single pulse)	(13.8 ps)	201
Dioxane	1	422 (BB)	XeCl (60 mJ, 35 ns)	$E = 22.1\%$	95
			N_2 (3.5 mJ, 15 ns)	$E = 22.0\%$	
Dioxane	1	410–430 (etalon)	Mode-locked YAG-TH (1 GW, 30 ps/pulse)	A few MW (25 ps) (synchronous pumping)	192
Dioxane	1.2	411–430 (grating) (osc + amp)	N_2 (1 MW, 10 ns, 50 Hz)	0.6 mJ	97

#M244 2'-Chloro-1,4-distyrylbenzene

| Toluene | | 420 (BB) | Glass-TH (1 MW) | | 202 |

#M245 4'-Chloro-1,4-distyrylbenzene

| Toluene | | 420 (BB) | Glass-TH (1 MW) | | 202 |

(continued)

Table 20 (continued)

Solvent	Concentration (mM)	Lasing wavelength (tuning) (nm)	Excitation	Output	Ref.
#M246 4,4'-Dichlor-1,4-distyrylbenzene					
Toluene		420 (BB)	Glass-TH (1 MW)		76
#M247 2'-Methoxy-1,4-distyrylbenzene					
Toluene		425 (BB)	Glass-TH (1 MW)		202
#M248 3'-Methoxy-1,4-distyrylbenzene					
Toluene		415 (BB)	Glass-TH (1 MW)		202
#M249 4'-Methoxy-1,4-distyrylbenzene					
Toluene		425 (BB)	Glass-TH (1 MW)		202
#M250 2,2"-Dimethoxy-1,4-distyrylbenzene					
Toluene		430 (BB)	Glass-TH (1 MW)		76

#M251 1-Styryl-4-[ω-vinyl-(n-biphenylyl)]benzene					
Toluene		432 (BB)	Glass-TH (1 MW)		76
#M252 1-Styryl-4-[ω-(2-naphthyl)-vinyl]benzene					
Toluene		425 (BB)	Glass-TH (1 MW)		202
Naphthalene (crystal)	10^{17} cm^{-3}	415 and 442 (BB) 4.2 K	Nd-THG (2 MW, 30 ns)	Thr = 0.07 J/cm^3	207
#M253 1,4-Bis(2-naphthyl)styrylbenzene					
Naphthalene (crystal)	10^{16} cm^{-3}	422 and 449 (BB) 4.2 K	Nd-THG (2 MW, 30 ns)	Thr = 5 mJ/cm^3	207
#M254 1,4-Bis(x-sulfostylyl)benzene					
Methanol	1-2	413-431	N$_2$	E = 1.7%	203
Water	1-2	415-443	N$_2$	E = 1.35%	203
#M255 1,4-Bis(x-sulfostyryl)-2-chlorobenzene					
Methanol	1-2	413-431	N$_2$	E = 2.8%	203

(continued)

Table 20 *(continued)*

Solvent	Concentration (mM)	Lasing wavelength (tuning) (nm)	Excitation	Output	Ref.
#M256 1,4-Bis(*p*-dimethylaminostyr-1)benzene					
PMMA	0.01-1	478 (BB)	Glass-TH (0.04 J, 40 ns)		168
#M257 1,4-Bis(*x,y*-dicyanostyryl)-2-chlorobenzene					
Dioxane	1-2	408-423	N$_2$	E = 1.9%	203
#M258 4,4'-Bis(*x,y*-dichlorostyryl)biphenyl					
Dioxane	1-2	416-437	N$_2$	E = 1.9%	203
#M259 4,4'-Bis(*x,y*-dicyanostyryl)biphenyl					
Dioxane	1-2	408-422	N$_2$	E = 1.95%	203
#M260 4,4'-Bis(2-sulfostyryl)biphenyl (disodium salt); stilbene 420; stilbene 3					
Methanol	1.8	408-453	N$_2$	E = 3.6%	203
Water	1.8	421-468		E = 2.6%	

Solvent	Conc.	Wavelength (nm)	Pump laser	Output	Ref.
Water + NP-10	1.8	416–455		E = 3.5%	
EG + methanol (9:1)	2	403–493 (BF filter)	Kr (UV all lines, 3.45 W)	660 mW, E = 19%	199
		420–472 (BF filter + etalon) (single axial mode, ring cavity)	Ar (351 and 363 nm, 2.5 W)	210 mW	84
EG	1.5	420–470 (tuning wedge)	Mode-locked Ar (351 nm, 141 mW, 130 ps)	(Syn-chronous pumping) 20 mW (1 ps) 60 mW (3.3–4.6 ps)	204
			(UV all lines, 400 mW, 300 ps)		
EG	0.88 g/l	406–480 (BF filter)	Ar or Kr (UV all lines, 3W)	500 mW, E = 18%	86
		415–460 (single axial mode)	Ar or Kr (UV all lines, 2.2 W)	40 mW	
Methanol + ethanol (1:1)	1.5	415–435 (grating)	YAG-TH (6–8 mJ, 8 ns)		94

(continued)

Table 20 *(continued)*

Solvent	Concentration (mM)	Lasing wavelength (tuning) (nm)	Excitation	Output	Ref.
		408–460 (grating) (osc + amp)	YAG–TH	E = 22%	98
Ethanol	1	405–467 (grating) (osc + amp)	XeCl (150 mJ, 10–20 ns)	E = 15%	26
EG	0.5	410–460 (grating) (osc + amp)	N_2 (1.5 MW, 4 ns)	E = 15%	
Water + ammonyx LO	0.5	425–470 (grating) (osc + amp)	N_2 (1.5 MW, 4 ns)		
EG + BZ		415–462 (single axial mode, ring cavity)	Ar (UV all lines, 4 W)	370 mW	303

	Solvent			
#M261 4,4'-Bis[[2-sulfo-4-(6,8-disulfo-2H-naphtho[2,1-d]triazol-2-yl)]styryl]benzene				
Methanol	1	485 (BB)	N_2 (1 MW, 2.5 ns)	155
#M262 2-Styrylbenzothiazole; uvitex RS; FBA 41				
Methanol		413-434 (prism)	N_2 (200 kW, 6 ns, 30 Hz)	198
#M263 Blankophor BP; FBA 116				
Methanol		412-468 (prism)	N_2 (200 kW, 6 ns, 30 Hz)	198
#M264 Tinopal RP; FBA 104				
Methanol		417-472 (prism)	N_2 (200 kW, 6 ns, 30 Hz)	198
#M265 Leukophor DC; FBA 69				
Methanol		447-508 (prism)	N_2 (200 kW, 6 ns, 30 Hz)	198
#M266 Uvitex SFC				
Methanol		409-459 (prism)	N_2 (200 kW, 6 ns, 30 Hz)	198

(continued)

Table 20 (continued)

Solvent	Concentration (mM)	Lasing wavelength (tuning) (nm)	Excitation	Output	Ref.
		#M267 Heliofor BDC			
Methanol		408–461 (prism)	N_2 (200 kW, 6 ns, 30 Hz)		198
		#M268 Uvitex NSI; FBA 65			
Methanol		410–463 (prism)	N_2 (200 kW, 6 ns, 30 Hz)		198
		#M269 1,4-Diphenylbutadiene			
Toluene	2.9	383 (BB)	Glass–TH (8 MW)	E = 1.5%	177
Cyclohexane	5	354–360	KrF	E = 10%	182
		#M270 1,1,4,4-Tetraphenylbutadiene			
Cyclohexane	1	501 (BB)	Ruby–SH (5 MW, 20 ns)	1 MW	164
Cumene	5	498 (−80 to 20°C, BB)	N_2 (2 ns)		204

423-438 (-130 to -70°C, BB)

[a]Chemical structures of conjugated diene compounds. The symbols (a)-(p) are shown in Table 21.

$R_1-CH=CH-R_2$

#M216; #M217; #M219- #M228

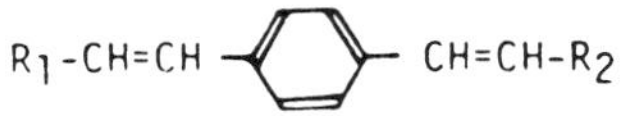

#M218

$R_1-CH=CH$—⬡—$CH=CH-R_2$

#M242- #M250; #M252- #M254; #M256; #M261

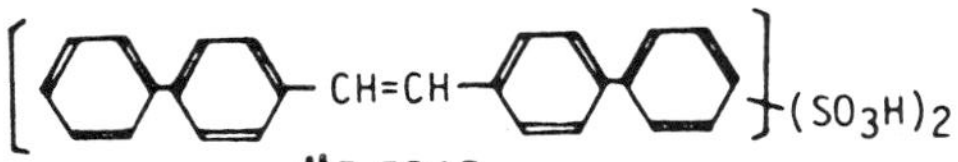

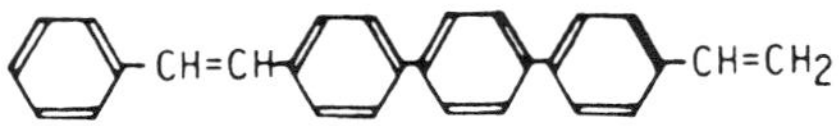

#M251

#M262

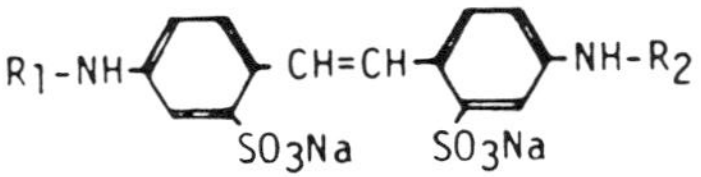

R_1-NH—⬡—$CH=CH$—⬡—$NH-R_2$
SO$_3$Na   SO$_3$Na

#M229- #M233

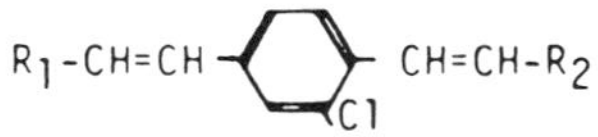

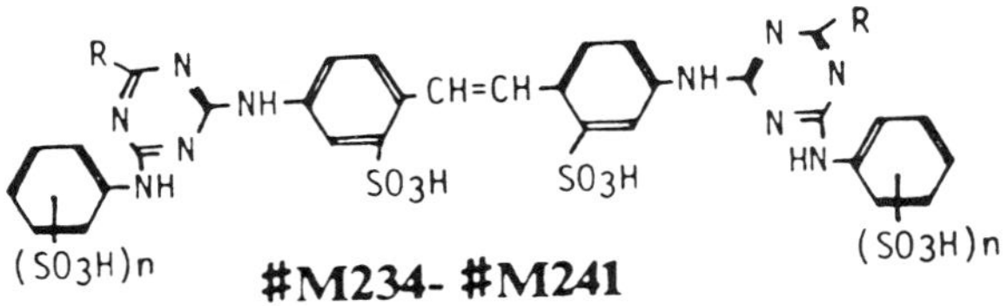

#M234- #M241

$R_1-CH=CH$—⬡—$CH=CH-R_2$
Cl

#M255; #M257

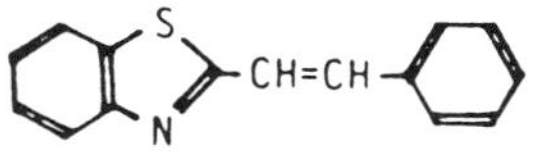

$R_1-CH=CH$—⬡—⬡—$CH=CH-R_2$

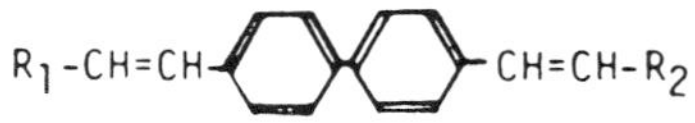

#M258- #M260

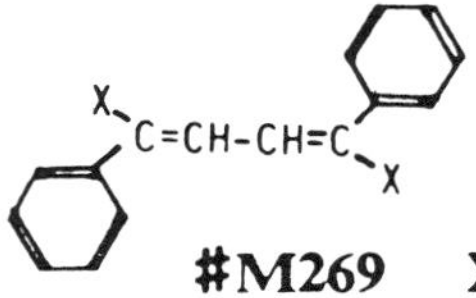

#M269   X=H
#M270   X=Ph

(continued)

Table 20 *(continued)*

Dye no.	R_1	R_2	Dye no.	R_1	R_2
#M216	Ph	(a)	#M231	(i)	(i)
#M217	(a)	(a)	#M232	(j) X = OH	(j) X = OH
#M219	(a)	(b)	#M233	(j) X = OCH_3	(j) X = OCH_3
#M220	(b)	(b)	#M234	R = OCH_3	n = 0
#M221	(c)	(c)	#M235	R = $N(C_2H_4OH)_2$	n = 0
#M222	(a)	(c)	#M236	R = $N(CH_2CHOH)_2$ | CH_3	n = 1
#M223	(b)	(c)			
#M224	Ph	(c)	#M237	R = $N(C_2H_4OH)_2$	n = 1
#M225	(d)	(d)			
#M226	Ph	(e) X = Ph	#M238	**R = N** $\overset{\textbf{CH}_3}{\underset{\textbf{C}_2\textbf{H}_4\textbf{OH}}{}}$	n = 1
#M227	Ph	(e) X = Na			
#M228	(f)	(f)			
#M229	(g)	(g)			
#M230	(h)	(h)	#M239	**R = N** (morpholino)	n = 2

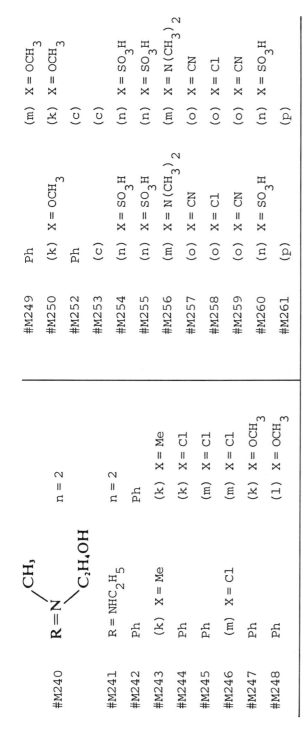

$$R = N \diagdown \begin{smallmatrix} CH_3 \\ C_2H_4OH \end{smallmatrix}$$

#M240			n = 2	#M249	Ph	(m) X = OCH$_3$
#M241	R = NHC$_2$H$_5$		n = 2	#M250	(k) X = OCH$_3$	(k) X = OCH$_3$
#M242	Ph		Ph	#M252	Ph	(c)
#M243	(k) X = Me		(k) X = Me	#M253	(c)	(c)
#M244	Ph		(k) X = Cl	#M254	(n) X = SO$_3$H	(n) X = SO$_3$H
#M245	Ph		(m) X = Cl	#M255	(n) X = SO$_3$H	(n) X = SO$_3$H
#M246	(m) X = Cl		(m) X = Cl	#M256	(m) X = N(CH$_3$)$_2$	(m) X = N(CH$_3$)$_2$
#M247	Ph		(k) X = OCH$_3$	#M257	(o) X = CN	(o) X = CN
#M248	Ph		(l) X = OCH$_3$	#M258	(o) X = Cl	(o) X = Cl
				#M259	(o) X = CN	(o) X = CN
				#M260	(n) X = SO$_3$H	(n) X = SO$_3$H
				#M261	(p)	(p)

177

Table 21. Abbreviations Used in Table 20

(a)

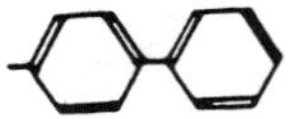

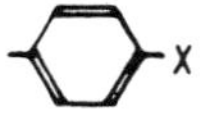

(b)

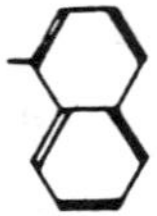

(c)

(d) SO_3K

(e) SO_3-x

(f) 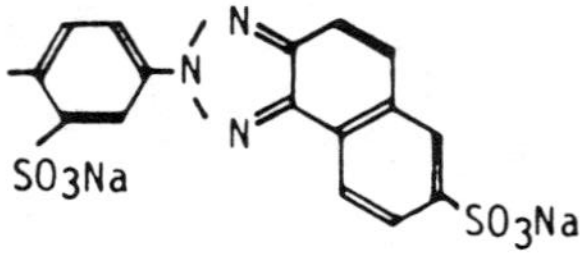 SO_3Na, SO_3Na

(g) $-CO-NH-$

(h) $-CH-NH-$, $N(C_2H_4OH)_2$

(i) $-C-NH_2$, $C-NH_2$

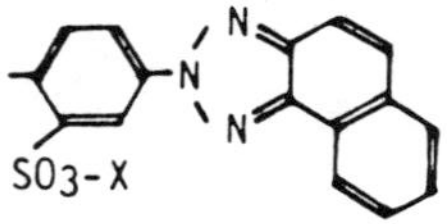

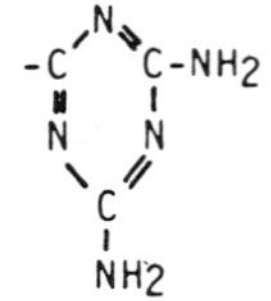

(î) x

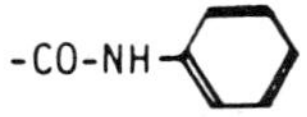

(j) 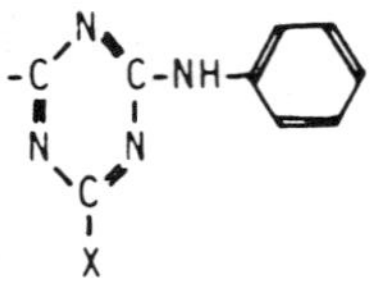 $-C-NH-$, $C-x$

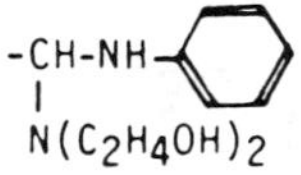

(k) 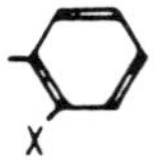 x

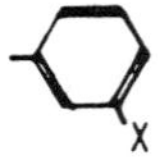

(m) x

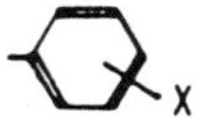

(n) x

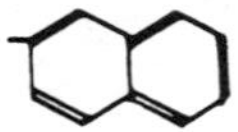

(o) x, x

(p) 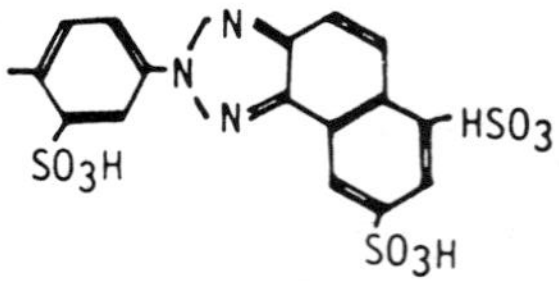 SO_3H, HSO_3, SO_3H

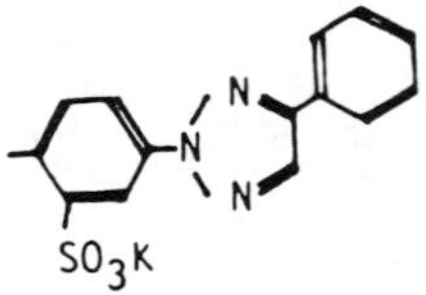

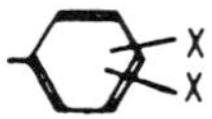

Table 22. Laser Characteristics of Miscellaneous Aromatic Compounds[a]

Solvent	Concentration (mM)	Lasing wavelength (tuning) (nm)	Excitation	Output	Ref.
#M271 Sodium salicylate					
Ethanol	>1	395–418 (grating)	N_2(100 kW, 10 ns, 100 Hz)		185
Ethanol	Satur.	403 (BB)	N_2 (530 kW, 3.5 ns)	E = 0.6%	139
#M272 Aminobenzoic acid					
Toluene		398–406 (grating)	N_2 (100 kW, 10 ns, 100 Hz)		185
#M273 2-(4-Biphenyl) indene; 4BPI					
DMF		388–393 (BB)	Fl (50 J, 200 ns, RT)	Thr = 40 J	184
DMF (deoxygenated)				Thr = 30 J	

(continued)

Table 22 (continued)

Solvent	Concentration (mM)	Lasing wavelength (tuning) (nm)	Excitation	Output	Ref.
#M274 Azulene					
Naphthalene (crystal)		398 (BB) 4.2 K	Nd-THG (2 MW, 30 ns)	Thr = 0.02 J/cm^2	207
#M275 Lachs					
Glycerin		540 (BB)	Ruby-SH		2
#M276 Fluorol 7GA; FBA 75; fluorol 555; green 10					
Methanol + HCl + COT	0.1 g/l (pH = 6)	530-608 (grating)	Fl (22 J)	15 mJ	206
Water + HCl + COT + ammonyx LO	0.13 g/l				

Methanol + coumarin 6 + COT (SA:DQOC) without SA	0.6 mg/l	535-590 (etalon)	Fl (260 J)	50 mJ (5 ps) (mode-locked) 150 mJ (1 µs)	205
Methanol	0.1	542-592 (grating)	Fl (150 ns, RT, 1 Hz)		87

^{a}Structures:

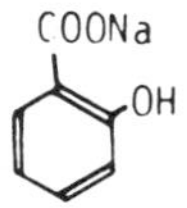

#M271   #M272   #M273   #M274   #M275* (Estimated)

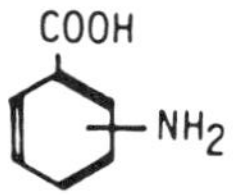

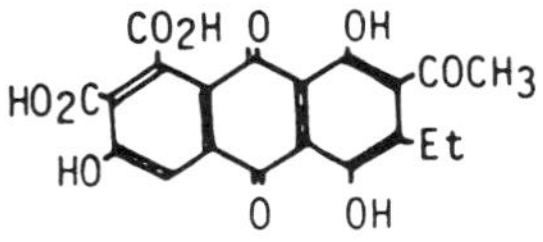

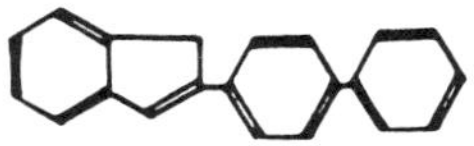

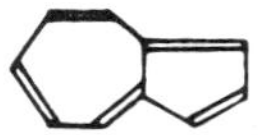

CHAPTER 6

Heterocyclic Compounds

Bicyclic compounds hold a majority in this class. Coumarin derivatives are particularly important. They are most effective and useful materials in the blue and green region. Quinolone derivatives are also efficient in the violet region. There are many reports on lasing of scintillator chemicals. They are composed of oxazole or oxadiazole derivatives, and show efficient lasing in the UV and violet region for short-pulse, UV-laser excitation.

I. Coumarin and Azacoumarin Derivatives

About a hundred coumarin derivatives (#M277–#M374 and #M542–#M546) have been developed after wide and systematical investigations. Figure 10a shows the structure of the coumarin ring (see Tables 23 and 24). In this compilation, they are arranged according to the substituent at the 7-position of this ring, because the substituent at this position most strongly affects its chemical characteristics. Usually, this position is occupied by a hydroxy, amino, or acetoxy radical.

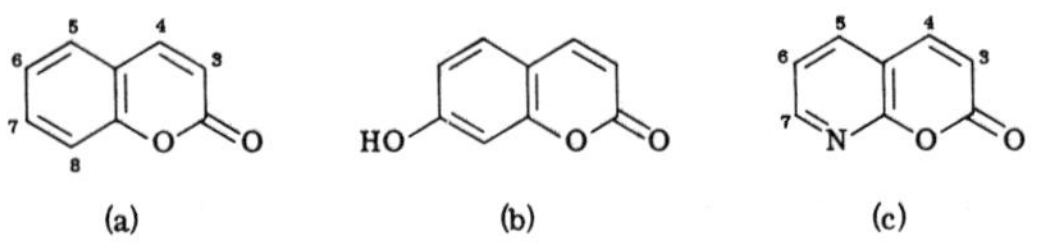

(a)   (b)   (c)

Fig. 10. Structures of (a) coumarin, (b) umbelliferone, and (c) azacoumarin.

7-Hydroxycoumarin is sometimes called umbelliferone (Fig. 10b). This type of compound has interesting lasing characteristics. For example, an acidic solution of 4-MU (#M281) forms a new fluorescence band whose maximum is at 490 nm. This was first explained by the emission from exciplex molecules with a proton, but after careful investigations, five different molecular states have been identified, when the solvent and/or the pH value are changed (215,241). Utilizing these different emission bands, the laser gain is obtained over a very wide region from 370 to 600 nm. In methyleneiminodiacetic acids such as #M291 and #M292, the lasing wavelengths depend not only on pH but also on the sort of metallic ions dissolved (154,219).

Systematic surveys on coumarin derivatives have been carried out by Eastman Kodak Company (83,165,223) and Schimitschek et al. (217,222,234). The lasing wavelengths of coumarin derivatives can be varied by the substitution, although the shift is rather small. Thus, a tunable range from 420 to 580 nm can be covered with the combination of #M311, #M330, #M337, and #M334, for example.

Coumarin compounds are as efficient as xanthene dyes. Even for the flashlamp with a long risetime, efficient lasing can be expected as well as for short-pulse pumping. The laser threshold for CW operation is low enough, although it requires a UV ion laser except for some of long-wavelength compounds like coumarine 6 (#M334).

A weak point of these coumarins is that chemical photobreaching is rapid compared with xanthene dyes. It is serious for flashlamp pumping. New fluorinated coumarins were developed to improve that (217). The photobreaching characteristics of many bicyclic compounds have been very widely investigated by the United States Naval Weapons Center (NWC) (265–269). The lasing wavelengths of azacoumarin derivatives (Fig. 10c) are generally longer than those of coumarin derivatives.

Eastman Kodak's catalog on laser chemicals lists coumarin 138, coumarin 338, and coumarin 339 (293). However, these compounds are not recorded in this compilation because no report on their lasing has been found.

II. Quinolone and Azaquinolone Derivatives

Figure 11 shows the structure of the quinolone-2 ring. Because this structure is similar to that of coumarins, the characteristics of quinolone derivatives (sometimes called "carbostyril") are also similar to those of coumarins, and their lasing efficiencies are fairly good (see Table 25). In comparison with the quinolone and coumarin derivatives with the same substituents, the former has a longer tunable range by 20–30 nm. Therefore, they are useful in the spectral region from 400 to 430 nm where laser action of coumarins is difficult. Azaquinolone (Fig. 11b) derivatives lase at wavelengths shorter than 400 nm.

A systematic survey of quinolone derivatives was carried out by Hammond et al. in NWC (184,249).

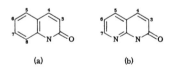

(a)   (b)

Fig. 11. Structures of (a) quinolone and (b) azaquinolone.

III. Oxazole and Benzoxazole Derivatives

Derivatives of furan, oxazole, and oxadiazole (Fig. 12) are known as scintillator materials for organic scintillation counters. Berlman collected and published the spectroscopic data on many of these compounds (270) (see Tables 26 and 27).

Usually the 2- and 5-positions of the oxazole ring are substituted by aryl radicals (139). The tunable range of these oxazole derivatives is from 330 to 450 nm. 2-Phenylbenzoxazole (#M435) is the shortest one (250). Because their fluorescence quantum yields are high, the lasing efficiency in short-pulse laser excitation is good; however, flashlamp pumping is quite difficult, and there is no report on the CW operation.

For vapor-phase dye lasers, these compounds are very important (271). They can lase under the vaporized condition at temperatures of 300–400°C by short-pulse excitation. POPOP (#M426) is only one material that showed laser action by electron-beam pumping (248). There is no successful report on the discharge-pumped vapor-phase dye laser (272).

IV. Oxadiazole Derivatives

Table 28 shows the oxadiazole derivatives that have an oxadiazole ring (Fig. 12b). The chemical and lasing characteristics and the wavelength region of this class of compounds are similar to those of oxazole derivatives. PBD (#M445) and its various substituents are well known, and their tunable ranges are in the shortest wavelength (~355 nm) pumpable by an N_2 laser.

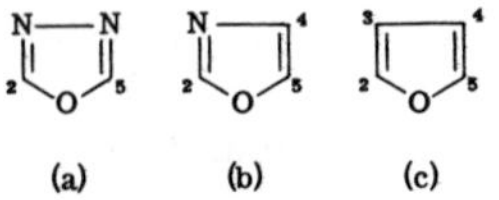

(a)   (b)   (c)

Fig. 12. Structures of (a) oxadiazole, (b) oxazole, and (c) furan.

V. Furan and Benzofuran Derivatives

Table 29 lists the furan (Fig. 12c) and benzofuran derivatives.

VI. Pyrazoline Derivatives

Table 30 lists the pyrazoline derivatives.

VII. Phthalimide and Naphthalimide Derivatives

The lasing region of phthalimide and naphthalimide compounds is in green and yellow (see Table 31). Flashlamp pumping is usable. In this case, it seems that the triplet quencher is effective. The efficiency of brilliant sulfoflavine (#486) is comparable with those of coumarins, even for flashlamp pumping.

VIII. Pteridine Derivatives

Table 32 shows the lasing characteristics of pteridine derivatives.

IX. Heterocyclic Salts

Heterocyclic salts listed in Tables 33 and 34 are classified as follows:

1. Phrylium salt   #M491–#M522
2. Thiapyrylium salt   #M524–#M527
3. Phosphorine   #M528–#M531
4. Pyridine   #M534–#M536 (and others)

Many pyrylium salts are known in the visible region, most of which were found by Basting et al. with N_2 laser pumping (155).

The structures of #M521 and #M522 do not correspond to the chemical names described in the paper (262). It seems that one of them is incorrect.

X. Miscellaneous Compounds

Table 35 lists miscellaneous compounds. The compounds from #M542 to #M546 should be listed in Table 23 of Section I (Coumarin and Azacoumarin Derivatives).

Table 23. Laser Characteristics of Coumarin and Azacoumarin Derivatives [a]

Solvent	Concentration (mM)	Lasing wavelength (tuning) (nm)	Excitation	Output	Ref.
#M277 6-Acetyl-5-hydroxy-4-methylcoumarin					
Ethanol + KOH		490 (BB)	Ruby-SH (2 MW, 40 ns)	Thr = 22 mJ	213
#M278 7-Hydroxycoumarin; umbelliferone					
Water	1	457 (BB)	Fl (1 µF, 20 kV, 700 ns, RT)		208
Water (basic)	1	458 (BB)	Fl (9J, 80 ns, RT)	Thr = 1.9 J	1
Alcohol	40 mg/l	405–429 (BB) 450–471 (BB, electric current)	N_2 (200 kW, 5 ns, 50 Hz)		209

(continued)

Table 23 (continued)

Solvent	Concentration (mM)	Lasing wavelength (tuning) (nm)	Excitation	Output	Ref.
		#M279 3-Cyanoumbelliferone			
Ethanol + water (7:3)		490–520 (grating)	Fl (85 J)	5 mJ	211
		#M280 3-Ethoxycarbonylumbelliferone; coumarin 15			
Water		465 (BB)	Fl (30 J)	Thr = 19 J	165
Ethanol + KOH		458 (BB)	Ruby-SH (2 MW, 40 ns)	Thr = 3.5 mJ	213
Ethanol		443 (BB)			
PMMA (thin film)	240		N$_2$ (140 kW)	Gain = 10 cm^{-1} (ASE)	212
Ethanol		410 (grating)	N$_2$ (70 kW)		211

190

#M281 4-Methylumbelliferone; 4-MU; coumarin 4; pilot 447

Water (pH > 9)	454 (BB)	Fl (100 J)	10 mJ (300 ns)	214
Ethanol + water (6:4)	437–544 (grating)	N$_2$ (100 kW, 100 Hz)		215
Ethanol + HCl (1/400, 0.1 M)	385–457 (grating)			
+ HCl (1/30, 0.1 M)	391–567 (grating)			
+ HCl (1/10, 1 M)	459–574 (grating)		48 kW	
Water	430–485 (grating)	Ruby-SH (5 MW, 15 ns)	100 kW	79
Ethanol (acid)	477–546 (grating + prism)	N$_2$ (130 kW)	5.7 kW	13

(continued)

Table 23 (continued)

Solvent	Concentration (mM)	Lasing wavelength (tuning) (nm)	Excitation	Output	Ref.
Water + NaOH	2	435–480 (prism)	Ar (351 and 364 nm, 3.3 W)	Thr = 482 mW	216
EG + benzyl alcohol (9:1)	~3	440–480 (BF filter)	Ar (351 and 364 nm, 1.5 W)		35
#M282 4-Trifluoromethylumbelliferone; C7F					
Ethanol + water (1:1)	0.75	506 (BB)	Fl (5 J)	0.6 kW	217
#M283 3-Cyano-4-methylumbelliferone					
Ethanol	2	399–475 (tuned)	N_2 (200 kW)		210
Ethanol + 16% water	2	440–510	N_2 (200 kW)		

Solvent	Conc.	Wavelength	Pump	Power/Energy	Ref.
Ethanol + 35% water	0.1	450–500	Fl (85 J)	15 mJ	
Water (base)	1	466–504 (tuned)	Ruby-SH (4.6 MW)	60 kW	211
Ethanol	1	405–451	Ruby-SH (2.5 MW)	37 kW	

#M284 3-Phenyl-4-methylumbelliferone

Solvent	Conc.	Wavelength	Pump	Power/Energy	Ref.
Ethanol + KOH		475 (BB)	Ruby-SH (2 MW, 40 ns)	Thr = 6 mJ	213
Alcohol		400–423 (BB)	N_2 (200 kW, 5 ns, 50 Hz)		209
		442–460 (BB, electric current)			

#M285 3-Iso-propyl-4-methylumbelliferone

Solvent	Conc.	Wavelength	Pump	Power/Energy	Ref.
Alcohol		426–447 (BB)	N_2 (200 kW, 5 ns, 50 Hz)		209
		452–471 (BB, electric current)			

(continued)

Table 23 (continued)

Solvent	Concentration (mM)	Lasing wavelength (tuning) (nm)	Excitation	Output	Ref.
		#M286 3-Ethyl-4-methylumbelliferone			
Water + KOH		458 (BB)	Ruby-SH (2 MW, 40 ns)	Thr = 4 mJ	213
Methanol		410 (BB)			
Ethanol		425 (BB)			
Ethanol + H_2SO_4		493 (BB)			
		#M287 3-n-Butyl-4-methylumbelliferone			
PMMA (thin film)	240		N_2 (140 kW)	Gain = 10 cm^{-1} (ASE)	212
		#M288 3-Benzyl-4-methylumbelliferone			
Ethanol or water (base)		463.5–468 (BB)	Fl (0.5 µF, 20 kV, 750 ns, RT)		78

Solvent	Conc.	Excitation	Emission (nm)	Ref.
Ethanol + NaOH	50 mg/l	Fl (200 J, 800 ns, RT)		74
#M289 3,4-Cyclopentenoumbelliferone				
Water (pH = 9)	2	Fl (0.3 μF, 1 μs)	Blue (BB)	218
#M290 4,8-Dimethylumbelliferone; 4,8-dimethyl-7-hydroxycoumarin				
Ethanol (base)	50 mg/l	Fl (0.3 μF, 25 kV, 500 ns, RT)	455–505 (grating)	99
#M291 7-Hydroxycoumarin-8-methyleneiminodiacetic acid; umbelliferone methyleneiminodiacetic acid				
Water (pH = 3.1)	5	N_2 (25 kW, 10 ns)	459 (BB)	154
Water (pH = 10)			469 (BB)	
+ Ca^{2+} (pH = 10.7)			470 (BB)	
+ Sr^{2+} (pH = 11)			471 (BB)	

(continued)

Table 23 *(continued)*

Solvent	Concentration (mM)	Lasing wavelength (tuning) (nm)	Excitation	Output	Ref.
+ Ba^{2+} (pH = 7.5)		473 (BB)			
+ Al^{3+} (pH = 3)		445 (BB)			
Water	0.25	453–464 (BB)	Fl (380 ns, RT)		
#M292 Calcein blue; 4-methylumbelliferone methyleneiminodiacetic acid					
Ethanol + NaOH	100 mg/l	459–464 (BB)	Fl (200 J, 0.5 µs, RT)		74
Water (pH = 9)	1	425–478 (grating)	N$_2$ (700 kW, 2.5 ns)		219
Water + Al^{3+} (pH = 5)	1	400–435 (grating)			
(pH = 9)		415–445 (grating)			

196

Solvent		Wavelength	Excitation		Ref.
(pH = 11)		430–450 (grating)			219
Water + Ba^{2+} (pH = 12)	1	435–478 (grating)			
Water + Sr^{2+} (pH = 5)		446 (BB)	N_2 (700 kW, 2.5 ns)		
+ Ca^{2+} (pH = 5)		446 (BB)			
#M293 6-Methoxyumbelliferone					
Water (pH = 9)	2	Blue (BB)	Fl (0.3 μF, 1 μs)		218
#M294 Esculin; 6-glucosyloxyumbelliferone					
Water			Fl (50 J, 400 ns)		102
Water (base)	1	469 (BB)	Fl (9 J, 80 ns, RT)	Thr = 1.3 J	1
Water		440–490 (prism) (ring cavity, single axial mode)	Fl (60 J)	4 kW	101

(continued)

Table 23 (continued)

Solvent	Concentration (mM)	Lasing wavelength (tuning) (nm)	Excitation	Output	Ref.
Methanol + NaOH	0.4	450–505 (grating)	Fl (86 J)	310 mJ (240 ns)	100
Ethanol	0.1	460 (BB)	Fl (100 J, 150 ns, RT)	300 mJ	186
			Fl (625 J, 800 ns, RT)	2.5 J, E = 0.4%	
Alcohol		423–441 (BB)	N$_2$ (200 kW, 5 ns, 50 Hz)		209
		460–478 (BB, electric current)			

#M295 5,7-Dihydroxy-4-methylcoumarin

Solvent	Concentration (mM)	Lasing wavelength (tuning) (nm)	Excitation	Output	Ref.
Ethanol + KOH		474 (BB)	Ruby-SH (2 MW, 40 ns)	Thr = 10 mJ	213

#M296 6,7-Dihydroxy-4-methylcoumarin

Solvent		Pump		Ref
Ethanol + KOH	471 (BB)	Ruby-SH (2 MW, 40 ns)	Thr = 48 mJ	213
Methanol	403 (BB)			
Ethanol + H_2SO_4	455 (BB)			

#M297 3-Biphenylyl-7-methoxycoumarin

Benzene	437 (BB)	N_2 (1 MW, 2.5 ns)		155

#M298 N-[4-(7-Methoxy-2H-2-oxo-1-benzopyran-3-yl)phenyl]-trimethylammonium methylsulfate

Water	457 (BB)	N_2 (1 MW, 2.5 ns)		155

#M299 1-(7-Methoxy-2H-2-oxo-1-benzopyran-3-yl)-3-methyl-1H-1,2,3-triazolium methylsulfate

Water	450 and 458 (BB)	N_2 (1 MW, 2.5 ns)		155

#M300 7-Methoxy-3-carbethoxycoumarin

Ethanol + KOH	459 (BB)	Ruby-SH (2 MW, 40 ns)	Thr = 13 mJ	213
Ethanol	422 (BB)			

(continued)

199

Table 23 (continued)

Solvent	Concentration (mM)	Lasing wavelength (tuning) (nm)	Excitation	Output	Ref.
#M301 7-Acetoxy-4-methylcoumarin					
Ethanol (base)	50 mg/1	441–486 (grating)	Fl (0.3 µF, 25 kV, 500 ns, RT)		99
Ethanol + KOH		457 (BB)	Ruby-SH (2 MW, 40 ns)	Thr = 6 mJ	213
Alcohol		400–420 (BB)	N_2 (200 kW, 5 ns, 50 Hz)	–	209
		440–465 (BB, electric current)			
#M302 7-Acetoxy-3-phenylcoumarin					
Ethanol + KOH		483 (BB)	Ruby-SH (2 MW, 40 ns)	Thr = 45 mJ	213

Compound	Solvent	Pump source	Wavelength (nm)	Ref.
#M303 7-Acetoxy-5-allyl-4,8-dimethylcoumarin	Ethanol (base) 50 mg/l	Fl (0.3 µF, 25 kV, 500 ns, RT) (grating)	458–515	99
#M304 7-Acetoxy-4-methyl-3-(α-naphthyl) coumarin	Ethanol + KOH	Ruby-SH (2 MW, 40 ns) Thr = 7 mJ	463 (BB)	213
#M305 7-Acetoxy-6-allyl-4,8-dimethylcoumarin	Ethanol 150 mg/l	Fl (200 J, 800 ns, RT)		74
#M306 7-Acetoxy-3-phenylcoumarin	Alcohol	N_2 (200 kW, 5 ns, 50 Hz) electric current	470–494 (BB)	209
#M307 7-Acetoxy-4-amyl-3-phenylcoumarin	Alcohol	N_2 (200 kW, 5 ns, 50 Hz) electric current	465–503 (BB)	209

(continued)

Table 23 (continued)

Solvent	Concentration (mM)	Lasing wavelength (tuning) (nm)	Excitation	Output	Ref.
#M308 7-Butyryloxy-4-methylcoumarin					
Water + acetonitrile (9:1) (pH = 9)	1	Blue (BB)	Fl (0.3 μF, 1 μs)		218
#M309 7-Aminocoumarin; C3H					
Ethanol	0.75	450 (BB)	Fl (5 J)	1 kW	222
#M310 7-Amino-3-phenylcoumarin; coumarin 10					
Water + DPA (4:1) + COT	1	470–500 (prism)	Ar (351 and 364 nm, 3.3 W)	Thr = 380 mW	216
#M311 7-Amino-4-methylcoumarin; coumarin 120; coumarin 440; blue 1					
Methanol		440 (BB)	Fl		83

Solvent		Wavelength (nm)	Pump source	Output	Ref.
Water + DPA (4:1) + COT	1	420–470 (prism)	Ar (351 and 364 nm, 3.3 W)	Thr = 608 mW	216
Ethanol	2.5	419–472 (grating)	N_2 (270 kW)	75 kW	220
EG + benzyl alcohol (9:1)	~3	424–477 (BF filter)	Ar (351 and 364 nm, 1.5 W)	120 mW	35
Methanol	0.2	425–470 (grating)	Fl (73 J)	150 mJ (240 ns)	100
Ethanol	0.7	441 (grating)	YAG-TH (10.5 MW, 8 ns, 20 Hz)	220 mWav.	221
Ethanol	8.7	440 (BB, short cavity)	Mode-locked glass-TH (1 mJ, 11 ps, single pulse)	(13.8 ps)	201
Ethanol		430 (BB)	Glass-TH (1–3 mJ, 6 ps)	0.2 mJ, E = 10% (ps pulse)	93
Ethanol	4	436 (BB)	XeCl (60 mJ, 35 ns)	E = 41.1%	95
Ethanol	5	420–475 (grating) (osc + amp)	N_2 (1 MW, 10 ns, 50 Hz)	0.8 mJ	97

(continued)

Table 23 (continued)

Solvent	Concentration (mM)	Lasing wavelength (tuning) (nm)	Excitation	Output	Ref.
#M312 7-Amino-4-trifluoromethylcoumarin; coumarin 151; coumarin 490; C3F; green 1					
Ethanol	0.75	484 (BB)	Fl (5 J)	5.0 kW	217
Ethanol + water (1:1)	0.75	496 (BB)	Fl (5 J)	5.5 kW	
Ethanol		490 (BB)	Fl (30 J, 1 μs)	Thr = 16 J	223
Methanol	0.2	470–508 (prism)	Fl (60 J)		224
Methanol + ammonyx LO	0.1	477–515 (grating)	Fl (150 ns, RT, 1 Hz)		87
#M313 7-Amino-4-methoxycoumarin					
Ethanol		417 (BB)	Fl (50 J, 200 ns, RT)	Thr = 30 J	184
#M314 7-Amino-3-ethyl-4-methylcoumarin					
Ethanol		438 (BB)	Ruby-SH (2 MW, 40 ns)	Thr = 7 mJ	213

#M315 7-Methylamino-4,6-dimethylcoumarin; coumarin 9

Solvent	Wavelength	Pump	Output	Ref
Ethanol	443 (BB)	Fl (3.6 μF, 10 kV, 1.2 μs, RT)		225
Ethanol (acid)	484 (BB)			
Ethanol	420–480 (grating)	N_2 (90 kW, 10 ns)	5 kW (2–7 ns)	226
Ethanol + HCl	435–525 (grating)			
Water + ethanol (2:1)	450–480 (etalon)	Fl (15 Hz, 450 Wav., 1.5 μs, RT)	288 mWav.	90

#M316 4-Methyl-7-sulfomethylaminocoumarin sodium salt; coumarin 175

Solvent	Wavelength	Pump	Output	Ref
Water	457 (BB)	Fl (30 J)	Thr = 14 J	165

#M317 3-Phenyl-7-sulfomethylaminocoumarin sodium salt; coumarin 316

Solvent	Wavelength	Pump	Output	Ref
Water	494 (BB)	Fl (30 J)	Thr = 16 J	165

#M318 7-(2-Hydroxyethylamino)-4-methylcoumarin; coumarin 360

Solvent	Wavelength	Pump	Output	Ref
Water	470 (BB)	Fl (30 J)	Thr = 14 J	165

(continued)

Table 23 (continued)

Solvent	Concentration (mM)	Lasing wavelength (tuning) (nm)	Excitation	Output	Ref.
#M319 7-Ethylamino-4-trifluoromethylcoumarin; coumarin 500					
Ethanol		500 (BB)	N_2		152
Ethanol	1	500 (BB)	KrF (0.2 J, 20 ns)	E = 18%	120
Ethanol	5	485–530 (grating)	YAG-TH (6–8 mJ, 8 ns)		94
Ethanol	10	473–547 (grating) (osc + amp)	N_2 (1 MW, 10 ns, 50 Hz)	1.2 mJ	97
		483–570 (grating) (osc + amp)	YAG-TH	E = 20%	98
Methanol + water		490–560 (grating)	Fl (10 Hz)	0.3 Wav. (1.4 μs)	126
Methanol + water + coumarin 504 (SA:DOCI)	0.055	505–520 (IF filter)	Fl (500 J)	100 μJ/ pulse (mode locking)	309

#M320 7-Ethylamino-4,6-dimethylcoumarin; coumarin 2; coumarin 450; blue 2

Solvent	Conc.	Tuning	Pump	Output	Ref.
Ethanol		446 (BB)	Fl (3.6 µF, 10 kV, 1.2 µs, RT)		225
Ethanol (acid)		487 (BB)			
Water + DPA(4:1)	2	430–480 (prism)	Ar (351 and 364 nm, 3.3 W)	Thr = 269 mW	216
EG + benzyl alcohol (9:1)	~3	430–492 (BF filter)	Ar (351 and 364 nm, 1.8 W)	168 mW	35
Methanol	0.2	430–485 (grating)	Fl (86 J)	270 mJ (240 ns)	100
Methanol	0.5	450 (BB)	Fl (484 J)	5 J, E = 1%	
Methanol	0.7	454 (grating)	YAG-TH (10.5 MW, 8 ns, 20 Hz)	330 mWav.	221
Ethanol	1	435–463 (grating)	YAG-TH (6–8 mJ, 8 ns)		94
EG	0.59 g/l	438–480 (BF filter)	Ar or Kr (UV all lines, 2 W)	320 mW, E = 15%	86

(continued)

Table 23 *(continued)*

Solvent	Concentration (mM)	Lasing wavelength (tuning) (nm)	Excitation	Output	Ref.
		432–480 (single axial mode)		36 mW	
Ethanol	10	428–465 (grating) (osc + amp)	N_2 (1 MW, 10 ns, 50 Hz)	0.85 mJ	97
Ethanol	5	427–480 (grating) (osc + amp)	XeCl (150 mJ, 10–20 ns)	E = 15%	26

#M321 7-Ethylamino-6-methyl-4-trifluoromethylcoumarin; coumarin 307; coumarin 503; green 3

Solvent	Concentration (mM)	Lasing wavelength (tuning) (nm)	Excitation	Output	Ref.
Ethanol		502 (BB)	Fl (30 J, 1 µs)	Thr = 12 J	223
PMMA (thin film)	240	500 (BB)	N_2 (140 kW)	Gain = 50 cm^{-1} (ASE)	212
		476.5 (DFB)			

Solvent	Conc.	Tuning range (mode)	Pump	Output	Ref.
Ethanol	7	476–542 (grating) (osc + amp)	XeCl (150 mJ, 10–20 ns)	$E = 14.2\%$	26
Ethanol	5	473–547 (grating) (osc + amp)	N_2 (1.5 MW, 4 ns)		
Methanol + ammonyx LO	0.1	481–540 (grating)	Fl (150 ns, RT, 1 Hz)		87
#M322 4-Methyl-7-(3-sulfopropyl) aminocoumarin sodium salt; coumarin 378					
Water		468 (BB)	Fl (30 J)	Thr = 11 J	165
#M323 4-Methyl-7-(4-sulfobutyl) aminocoumarin sodium salt; coumarin 380					
Water		470 (BB)	Fl (30 J)	Thr = 11 J	165
#M324 7-Dimethylaminocoumarin; C2H					
Ethanol	0.75	465 (BB)	Fl (5 J)	7.5 kW	222
#M325 7-Dimethylamino-3-ethoxycarbonylcoumarin; coumarin 14					
Ethanol			Fl (30 J, 1 µs)		223
Ethanol	0.2	(Prism)	Fl (750 J)	3.8 J, $E = 0.5\%$	125

(continued)

Table 23 (continued)

Solvent	Concentration (mM)	Lasing wavelength (tuning) (nm)	Excitation	Output	Ref.
#M326 7-Dimethylamino-4-methylcoumarin; coumarin 311					
Ethanol		453 (BB)	Fl (50 J, 200 ns, RT)	Thr = 12 J	184
PMMA (thin film)		(BB)	N_2 (140 kW)	Gain = 13 cm^{-1} (ASE)	212
#M327 7-Dimethylamino-4-trifluoromethylcoumarin; coumarin 152; coumarin 485; C2F; green 6					
Ethanol	0.75	519 (BB)	Fl (5 J)	2.0 kW	217
Dioxane	0.75	479 (BB)	Fl (5 J)	6.1 kW	
Ethanol		520 (BB)	Fl (30 J, 1 μs)	Thr = 30 J	223
Ethanol	1.3–10	520 (grating + etalon)	YAG-TH (120 mJ, 5–6 ns, 10 Hz)	16 mJ, E = 19%	227
Ethanol	10	490–562 (grating) (osc + amp)	N_2 (1 MW, 50 Hz, 10 ns)	1 mJ	97

Solvent	Conc.	Tuning range	Pump	Output	Ref.
Ethanol	7.7	503–570 (grating) (osc + amp)	YAG–TH	E = 16%	98
		490–570 (grating) (osc + amp)	XeCl (150 mJ, 10–20 ns)	E = 5.5%	26

#M328 7-Diethylamino-4-hydroxy-3-methylcoumarin

Solvent	Conc.	Tuning range	Pump	Output	Ref.
Ethanol		429–442 (BB)	Nd–THG		228
Water + 1N HCl		451–466 (BB)			

#M329 7-Diethylaminocoumarin; LD 466; C1H; blue 4

Solvent	Conc.	Tuning range	Pump	Output	Ref.
Ethanol	0.75	466 (BB)	Fl (5 J)		222
Ethanol	1	450–485 (grating)	YAG–TH (6–8 mJ, 8 ns)		94
Methanol + ammonyx LO	0.08	462–490 (grating)	Fl (150 ns, RT, 1 Hz)		87

#M330 7-Diethylamino-4-methylcoumarin; DAMC; 7D4MC; coumarin 1; coumarin 460; blue 3; pilot 449

Solvent	Conc.	Tuning range	Pump	Output	Ref.
Ethanol		460 (BB)	Fl		229

(continued)

Table 23 (continued)

Solvent	Concentration (mM)	Lasing wavelength (tuning) (nm)	Excitation	Output	Ref.
Ethanol		460.7 (grating)	Fl	300 kW	230
Ethanol	0.1	460 (BB)	Fl (3.6 μF, 20 kV)	(Active mode locking)	231
		445–490 (grating)	N_2 (120 kW, 10 ns, 100 Hz)	E = 27%	130
Ethanol	1–10	438.5–482 (BB, concentration)	N_2 (20–40 kW)	E = 20%	232
Ethanol	2	445–475 (grating)	Ruby-SH (5 MW, 15 ns)	7 kW	79
	0.25	(BB)	Fl (600 J, 400 ns, RT)	4.18 J (600 ns), E = 0.7%	233
EG + benzyl alcohol (9:1)	~3	445–505 (BF filter)	Ar (351 and 364 nm, 1.35 W)	166 mW	35

Solvent	Conc.	Tuning range (nm)	Pump	Output	Ref.
Ethanol	0.7	457 (grating)	YAG–TH (10.5 MW, 8 ns, 20 Hz)	380 mWav., E = 22%	221
Ethanol	7.1–59	450–465 (short cavity)	Mode-locked glass–TH (11 ps, 1 mJ, single pulse)	40 µJ, 13.8 ps	201
Ethanol	0.15–3	456–463 (BF filter)	Xe (365 nm, 5 kW, 200 ns, 10 Hz)	1 kW, E = 20% (120 ns)	195
Ethanol	5	440–475 (grating)	YAG–TH (6–8 mJ, 8 ns)		94
Ethanol	4	456 (BB)	XeCl (60 mJ, 35 ns)	E = 35.4%	95
EG	1.8 g/l	450–500 (BF filter)	Ar or Kr (UV all lines, 2.5 W)	370 mW, E = 15%	86
		450–500 (single axial mode)	Ar or Kr (UV all lines, 2 W)	32 mW	
Ethanol	10	440–478 (grating) (osc + amp)	N_2 (1 MW, 10 ns, 50 Hz)	1 mJ	97
Ethanol		443–490 (grating) (osc + amp)	YAG–TH	E = 12%	98

(continued)

Table 23 (continued)

Solvent	Concentration (mM)	Lasing wavelength (tuning) (nm)	Excitation	Output	Ref.
#M331 7-Diethylamino-3-ethyl-4-methylcoumarin					
Ethanol		463 (BB)	Ruby-SH (2 MW, 40 ns)	Thr = 2 mJ	213
#M332 2-(7-Diethylamino-2H-2-oxo-1-benzopyran-3-yl)-1,3-dimethylbenzimidazolium chloride					
Methanol	Satur.	508 (BB)	N_2 (1 MW, 2.5 ns)		155
#M333 7-Diethylamino-4-trifluoromethylcoumarin; coumarin 35; coumarin 481; pilot 481; ClF; blue 7					
Dioxane	0.75	481 (BB)	Fl (5 J, 20 Hz)	3.8 kW	234
Dioxane	0.7	489 (grating)	YAG-TH (10.5 MW, 8 ns, 20 Hz)	390 mWav., E = 23%	221
Dioxane	5	465-510 (grating)	YAG-TH (6-8 mJ, 8 ns)		94
Dioxane	10	465-516 (grating)	N_2		236

Ethanol	10	492–545 (grating)			
Dioxane + ethanol (2:1)	10	480–541 (grating)			
Dioxane or cyclohexane	3.6	481 (BB)	KrF (160 mJ, 0.2 Wav.)	11.4 mJ (10–12 ns)	190
Dioxane	10	460–517 (grating) (osc + amp)	N_2 (1 MW, 10 ns, 50 Hz)	1.2 mJ	97
Dioxane	0.15	475–490 (grating)	Fl (150 ns, RT, 1 Hz)		87

#M334 3-(2-Benzothiazolyl)-7-diethylaminocoumarin; coumarin 6; green 8; coumarin 540

Methanol		540 (BB)	Fl		83
Water + DPA (4:1) + ammonyx LO + COT	0.3	515–585 (prism)	Ar (488 nm, 1.5 W)	220 mW, Thr = 174 mW	216
Benzyl alcohol	~3	516–567 (BF filter)	Ar (488 nm, 2.3 W)	196 mW	35

(continued)

Table 23 *(continued)*

Solvent	Concentration (mM)	Lasing wavelength (tuning) (nm)	Excitation	Output	Ref.
Ethanol	0.1	540 (BB)	Fl (100 J, 150 ns, RT)	60 mJ	186
Methanol	0.2	520–560 (grating)	Fl (73 J)	170 mJ (240 ns)	100
Ethanol	10	507–529 (grating)	N_2^+ (478 nm, 1 mJ, 250 kW, 10 Hz)		235
Ethanol	Satur.	528 (BB)	XeCl (60 mJ, 35 ns)	E = 20.4%	95
Ethanol		515–575 (BF filter + etalon) (ring cavity, single axial mode)	Ar (6 W, 488 nm)	490 mW	84
Benzyl alcohol + glycerin (4:1)	0.68 g/l	520–580 (BF filter) 520–570 (single axial mode)	Ar (488 nm, 3 W)	370 mW, E = 13% 90 mW	86

Solvent	Conc.	Tuning range (nm)	Pump	Output	Ref.
Glycerin + alcohol + COT		510–546 (single axial mode, ring cavity)	Ar (488 nm, 6 W)	350 mW	303

#M335 3-(5-Chloro-2-benzothiazolyl)-7-diethylaminocoumarin; coumarin 34

Solvent	Conc.	Tuning range (nm)	Pump	Output	Ref.
Ethanol		540 (BB)	Fl	Thr = 10.2 J	143

#M336 3-(2-Benzimidazolyl)-7-diethylaminocoumarin; coumarin 7; coumarin 535

Solvent	Conc.	Tuning range (nm)	Pump	Output	Ref.
Water + DPA (4:1) + ammonyx LO + COT	0.4	500–575 (prism)	Ar (477 nm, 800 mW)	80 mW, Thr = 148 mW	216
Benzyl alcohol	~3	495–567 (BF filter)	Ar (477 nm, 1.2 W)	117 mW	35
Ethanol		524 (BB)	Fl	Thr = 9.9 J	143

#M337 7-Diethylamino-3-(1-methyl-2-benzimidazolyl)coumarin; coumarin 30; coumarin 515

Solvent	Conc.	Tuning range (nm)	Pump	Output	Ref.
Methanol		510 (BB)	Fl		83
Water + DPA (4:1) + COT	1	495–515 (prism)	Ar (458 nm, 370 mW)	Thr = 443 mW	216

(continued)

217

Table 23 *(continued)*

Solvent	Concentration (mM)	Lasing wavelength (tuning) (nm)	Excitation	Output	Ref.
Benzyl alcohol	~3	492–550 (BF filter)	Ar (458 nm, 0.8 W)		35
Methanol	0.2	480–525 (grating)	Fl (73 J)	100 mJ (240 ns)	100
Ethanol	10	482–507 (grating)	N_2^+ (428 nm, 1 mJ, 250 kW, 10 Hz)		235
EG	0.24 g/l	480–545 (BF filter)	Kr (all violet lines, 2.5 W)	290 mW, E = 13%	86
		480–540 (single axial mode)		40 mW	
EG + BZ		485–530 (single axial mode)	Kr (all violet lines, 4.6 W)	380 mW	303

#M338 4-Methyl-7-[*N*-methyl-*N*-(4-sulfobutyl)amino]-coumarin sodium salt; coumarin 306

Solvent	Concentration (mM)	Lasing wavelength (tuning) (nm)	Excitation	Output	Ref.
Water		478 (BB)	Fl (30 J)	Thr = 43 J	165

#M339 4-Methyl-7-bis(3-sulfopropyl) aminocoumarin disodium salt; coumarin 379

Water		473 (BB)	Fl (30 J)	Thr = 15 J	165

#M340 7-Bis(4-sulfobutyl)amino-4-methylcoumarin disodium salt; coumarin 381

Water		478 (BB)	Fl (30 J)	Thr = 25 J	165

#M341 7-(3-Chloro-5-diethylaminotriazin-2-yl)amino-3-phenylcoumarin

Methanol	1	446 (BB)	N_2 (1 MW, 2.5 ns)		155

#M342 Piperidino[3,2-g]coumarin; C4H

Ethanol	0.75	477 (BB)	Fl (5 J)	5.0 kW	222

#M343 N-Methylpiperidino[3,2-g]coumarin; C8H

Ethanol	0.75	475 (BB)	Fl (5 J)	7 kW	222

#M344 4-Trifluoromethylpiperidino[3,2-g]coumarin; coumarin 340; C4F

Ethanol	0.75	522 (BB)	Fl (5 J)	6.2 kW	217
Ethanol		513 (BB)	Fl (30 J, 1 μs)	Thr = 12 J	223

(continued)

Table 23 *(continued)*

Solvent	Concentration (mM)	Lasing wavelength (tuning) (nm)	Excitation	Output	Ref.
#M345 *N*-Methyl-4-trifluoromethylpiperidino[3,2-*g*]coumarin; coumarin 522; C8F; green 7					
Ethanol	0.75	522 (BB)	Fl (5 J)	7.8 kW	217
Ethanol	5	505-550 (grating)	YAG-TH (6-8 mJ, 8 ns)		94
Methanol + ammonyx LO	0.2	501-568 (grating)	Fl (150 ns, RT, 1 Hz)		87
Ethanol (SA:DASBTI)	0.25	508-524 (etalon)	Fl (100 J)	4 MW, 4 ps (mode locking)	307
#M346 *N*-Ethyl-4-trifluoromethylpiperidino[3,2-*g*]coumarin; coumarin 355					
Ethanol		522 (BB)	Fl (30 J, 1 µs)	Thr = 11 J	223

#M347 4-Methyl-N-(3-sulfopropyl)piperidino[3,2-g]coumarin
      sodium salt; coumarin 386

Solvent					
Water	486 (BB)	Fl (30 J)		Thr = 10 J	165

#M348 4-Methyl-N-(4-sulfobutyl)piperidino[3,2-g]couamrin
      sodium salt; coumarin 388

Water	489 (BB)	Fl (30 J)		Thr = 10 J	165

   #M349 4-Trifluoromethylpiperidino[2,3-h]coumarin; C5F

Ethanol	521 (BB)	Fl (5 J)	0.75	1.3 kW	217

#M350 N-Methyl-4-trifluoromethylpiperidino[2,3-h]coumarin; C9F

Ethanol	537 (BB)	Fl (5 J)	0.75	6.8 kW	217

#M351 1,2,4,5-3H,6H,10H-Tetrahydro[1]benzopyrano[9,9a,1-gh]-
      quinolizin-10-one; C6H; LD 490; green 2

Ethanol	490 (BB)	Fl (5 J)	0.75	7 kW	222
Methanol	459-525 (prism)	Fl (80 J)	0.2	350 mJ (300 ns)	224
		Cavity dumping		300 mJ (20 ns)	

(continued)

221

Table 23 *(continued)*

Solvent	Concentration (mM)	Lasing wavelength (tuning) (nm)	Excitation	Output	Ref.
Methanol + water		470–500 (grating)	Fl (10 Hz)	0.8 Wav., (1.4 µs)	126
Methanol + ammonyx LO	0.1	465–529 (grating)	Fl (150 ns, RT, 1 Hz)		87
#M352 2,3,5,6-1H,4H-Tetrahydro-8-methylquinolazino[9,9a,1-gh] coumarin; coumarin 102; coumarin 480; blue 6					
Methanol		480 (BB)	Fl		83
HFIP		510 (BB)			
Water + DPA (4:1)	2	465–500 (prism)	Ar (351 and 364 nm, 3.3 W)	Thr = 323 mW	216
Ethanol	0.75	480 (BB)	Fl (5 J)	4.1 kW	234
EG + benzyl alcohol (9:1)	~3	460–522 (BF filter)	Ar (351 and 364 nm, 1.5 W)	106 mW	35

Solvent		λ (nm)	Pump	Output	Ref.
Methanol	0.7	485 (grating)	YAG-TH (10.5 MW, 8 ns, 20 Hz)	270 mWav.	221
Ethanol		480 (BB)	Fl (30 J, 1 μs)	Thr = 12 J	223
Methanol	0.2	460–525 (grating)	Fl (86 J)	400 mJ (240 ns)	100
Ethanol	10	453–510 (grating)	N_2^+ (428 nm, 1 mJ, 250 kW, 10 Hz)		235
		470 (BB)	Mode-locked glass–TH (1–3 mJ, 6 ps, single pulse)	0.3 mJ, E = 15% (12 ps)	93
Methanol (SA:DOC)	0.22	475–490 (etalon)	Fl	Mode locked (10 ps)	237
Ethanol	4	474.5 (BB)	XeCl (60 mJ, 35 ns)	E = 39.8%	95
Ethanol	10	453–495 (grating) (osc + amp)	N_2 (1 MW, 10 ns, 50 Hz)	0.9 mJ	97
		460–510 (grating) (osc + amp)	YAG–TH	E = 13%	98

(continued)

223

Table 23 (continued)

Solvent	Concentration (mM)	Lasing wavelength (tuning) (nm)	Excitation	Output	Ref.
Ethanol	6	456–503 (grating) (osc + amp)	XeCl (150 mJ, 10–20 ns)	E = 18.5%	26
EG + BZ		460–519 (ring cavity, single axial mode)	Kr (violet 4.8 W)	0.58 W	303
Ethanol		474.5 (BB)	XeCl (3 J)	1.1 J, E = 37%	306

#M353 2,3,5,6-1H,4H-Tetrahydro-8-trifluoromethylquinolizino[9,9a,1-gh] coumarin; coumarin 153; coumarin 540A; pilot 495; C6F; green 9

Solvent	Concentration (mM)	Lasing wavelength (tuning) (nm)	Excitation	Output	Ref.
Ethanol		543 (BB)	Fl	Thr = 12.6 J	143
Ethanol	0.75	538 (BB)	Fl (5 J)	6 kW	217
Dioxane	10	507 (grating)	N_2		236

224

Solvent	Range (nm)	Pump	Output	Ref
Ethanol	519–575 (grating + etalon) (single axial mode)	N$_2$ (50 kW, 3 ns, 30 Hz)	8 kW	238
Ethanol	513–580 (grating) (osc + amp)	XeCl (150 mJ, 10–20 ns)	E = 8.4%	26
Ethanol	516–592 (grating) (osc + amp)	N$_2$ (1.5 MW, 4 ns)		
Methanol	520–586 (grating)	Fl (150 ns, RT, 1 Hz)		87
Ethanol	518–547 (etalon)	Fl (100 J)	3 MW, 3.5 ps (mode locking)	308

#M354 2,3,6,7,10,11-Hexahydro-1H,5H,9H-quinolizine[1,9-gh]cyclopenta[c]coumarin; coumarin 106; coumarin 478

Solvent	Range (nm)	Pump	Output	Ref
Ethanol	478 (BB)	Fl (30 J, 1 μs)	Thr = 13 J	223

(continued)

225

Table 23 (continued)

Solvent	Concentration (mM)	Lasing wavelength (tuning) (nm)	Excitation	Output	Ref.
	#M355	9-Acetyl-1,2,4,5,3H,6H,10H-tetrahydro-1-benzopyrano[9,9a,1-gh]-quinolizin-10-one; coumarin 334; coumarin 521			
Ethanol		521 (BB)	Fl (30 J, 1 μs)	Thr = 12 J	223
	#M356	9-Cyano-1,2,4,5,3H,6H,10H-tetrahydro-1-benzopyrano[9,9a,1-gh]-quinolizin-10-one; coumarin 337; coumarin 523			
Ethanol		522 (BB)	Fl (30 J, 1 μs)	Thr = 12 J	223
	#M357	9-Carboxy-1,2,4,5,3H,6H,10H-tetrahydro-1-benzopyrano[9,9a,1-gh]-quinolizin-10-one; coumarin 343; coumarin 519; green 5			
Ethanol		519 (BB)	Fl (30 J, 1 μs)	Thr = 12 J	223
Water		518 (BB)	Fl (30 J)	Thr = 8 J	165
Methanol	0.2	490–513 (grating)	Fl (150 ns, RT)		87

#M358 1,2,4,5-3H,6H,10H-Tetrahydro-9-carbethoxy-1-benzopyrano[9,9a,1-gh]-quinolizin-10-one; coumarin 314; coumarin 504; green 4

Ethanol		506 (BB)	Fl	Thr = 10.9 J	143
Ethanol		504 (BB)	Fl (30 J, 1 μs)	Thr = 8 J	223
Glycerin + water + coumarin 6 (SA:PIC)	0.25	520 (etalon)	Fl (500 J)	3 mJ (10 ps) (mode locked)	
Methanol + ammonyx LO	0.1	484-537 (grating)	Fl (150 ns, RT, 1 Hz)		87
Methanol + water		489-520 (grating)	Fl (10 Hz)	0.95 Wav. (1.4 μs)	126

#M359 (1,2,4,5,3H,6H,10H-Tetrahydro-10-oxo-[1]benzopyrano[9,9a,1-gh]-quinolizin-8-yl)acetic acid; coumarin 217

Water		514 (BB)	Fl (30 J)	Thr = 9 J	165

#M360 3-Phenyl-7-(4-phenylpyrazol-1-yl) coumarin

Benzene	1	434 (BB)	N_2 (1 MW, 2.5 ns)		155

#M361 7-(4-Methyl-5-phenyl-2H-1,2,3-triazol-2-yl)-3-phenylcoumarin

Benzene	1	434 (BB)	N_2 (1 MW, 2.5 ns)		155

(continued)

227

Table 23 *(continued)*

Solvent	Concentration (mM)	Lasing wavelength (tuning) (nm)	Excitation	Output	Ref.
#M362 7-(4-Ethyl-5-methyl-2H,1,2,3-triazol-2-yl)-3-(1H,1,2,4-triazol-1-yl)coumarin					
Benzene	1	414 (BB)	N$_2$ (1 MW, 2.5 ns)		155
#M363 7-(4-Methyl-5-phenyl-2H,1,2,3-triazol-2-yl)-3-(1H,1,2,4-triazol-1-yl)coumarin					
Benzene	1	426 (BB)	N$_2$ (1 MW, 2.5 ns)		155
Dichloro-methane	1	430 (BB)			
#M364 3-p-Tolyl-7-(1H,1,2,3-triazol-1-yl)coumarin					
Benzene	1	421 (BB)	N$_2$ (1 MW, 2.5 ns)		155
#M365 3-p-Tolyl-7-(1H,1,2,4-triazol-1-yl)coumarin					
Benzene	1	423 (BB)	N$_2$ (1 MW, 2.5 ns)		155

#M366 7-(3,5-Dimethyl-1H,1,2,4-triazol-1-yl)-3-(p-methoxyphenyl)coumarin

Benzene	1	438 (BB)	N_2 (1 MW, 2.5 ns)	155

#M367 1-[7-(4-Chloro-3-methyl-pyrazol-1-yl)-2H-2-oxo-1-benzopyran-3-yl]-4-methyl-1,2,4-triazolium methylsulfate

Methanol	1	458 (BB)	N_2 (1 MW, 2.5 ns)	155

#M368 5-n-Butoxy-6-methyl-2-[3-(4-chloropyrazol-1-yl)-2H-2-oxo-1-benzopyran-7-yl]benzotriazolium inner salt

Benzene	1	439	N_2 (1 MW, 2.5 ns)	155

#M369 3-[7-(5-Ethyl-4-methyl-2H,1,2,3-triazol-2-yl)-2H-2-oxo-1-benzopyran-3-yl]-1-methyl-3H,1,3,4-triazolium methylsulfate

Water	1	467 (BB)	N_2 (1 MW, 2.5 ns)	155

#M370 3-Methyl-1-(3-tolyl-2H-2-oxo-1-benzopyran-7-yl)-1H,1,2,3-triazolium methylsulfate

Methanol	1	502 (BB)	N_2 (1 MW, 2.5 ns)	155

#M371 Coumarin 24

Methanol		510 (BB)	F1	60

(continued)

Table 23 (continued)

Solvent	Concentration (mM)	Lasing wavelength (tuning) (nm)	Excitation	Output	Ref.
#M372 Coumarin 445					
Ethanol		445 (BB)	Fl		152
EG		435–484	Ar (CW)		126
Methanol + water		420–460 (grating)	Fl (10 Hz)	0.5 Wav. (1.4 µs)	
#M373 Coumarin 527					
Ethanol		527 (BB)	N_2		152
#M374 Coumarin 531					
Ethanol		531 (BB)	N_2		152
#M375 7-Hydroxy-4-methyl-8-azacoumarin					
Ethanol		431 (BB)	Fl (50 J, 200 ns, RT)	Thr = 18 J	184

#M376 7-Amino-3,4-dimethyl-8-azacoumarin

Solvent	Conc.	Wavelength	Pump		Ref.
Ethanol	5	(BB)	N_2 (10 ns, 20 kW, 10 Hz)		184

#M377 7-Dimethylamino-4-methyl-8-azacoumarin

Solvent	Conc.	Wavelength	Pump		Ref.
Ethanol		434 (BB)	Fl (50 J, 200 ns, RT)	Thr = 20 J	184
			Fl (70 J, 400–600 ns, RT)	Thr = 65 J	

#M378 7-Morpholino-4-methyl-8-azacoumarin; LD 425; violet 3

Solvent	Conc.	Wavelength	Pump		Ref.
Ethanol		431 (BB)	Fl (50 J, 200 ns, RT)	Thr = 18 J	184
Methanol	0.2	419–440 (grating)	Fl (150 ns, RT, 1 Hz)		87
Dioxane	7.5	404–425	N_2		152
Ethanol	3	408–448			

#M379 8-Aza-4-trifluoromethyl(1,4-dimethylpiperidino)[3,2-g]coumarin; AC2F

Solvent	Conc.	Wavelength	Pump		Ref.
Ethanol	0.75	490 (BB)	Fl (5 J)	9.0 kW	222

(continued)

Table 23 (continued)

Solvent	Concentration (mM)	Lasing wavelength (tuning) (nm)	Excitation	Output	Ref.
	#M380 8-Aza-4-trifluoromethyl(1,2,4-trimethylpiperidino)-[3,2-g]coumarin; AC3F; green 2.5				
Methanol	0.2	465–511 (prism)	Fl (80 J)		224
Methanol + ammonyx LO	0.08	471–525 (grating)	Fl (150 ns, RT, 1 Hz)		87

[a] Chemical structures of coumarin and azacoumarin derivatives. The numbers (1)–(19) are shown in Table 24.

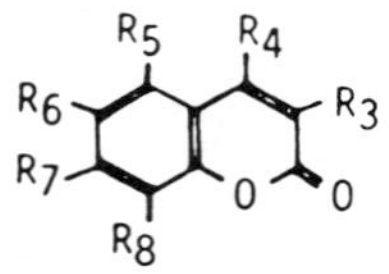

#M277- #M288; #M290- #M307; #M315; #M320; #M321

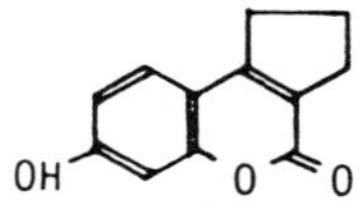

#M289

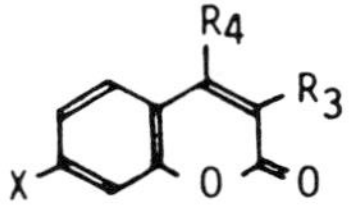

#M308- #M314; #M316- #M319; #M322- #M341; #M360- #M370

232

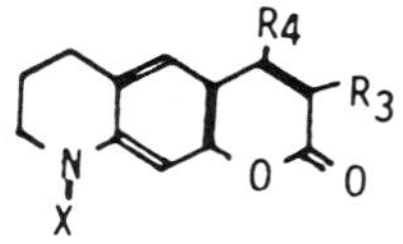

#M342- #M348

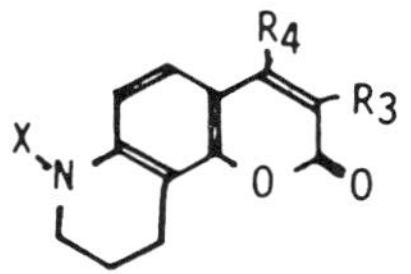

#M349; #M350

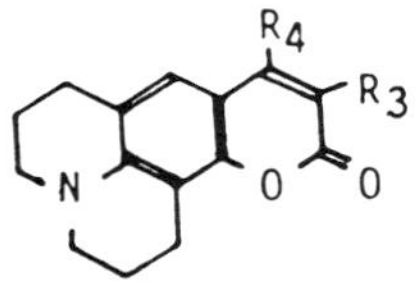

#M351- #M353; #M355- #M359

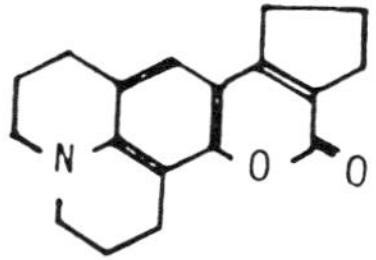

#M354

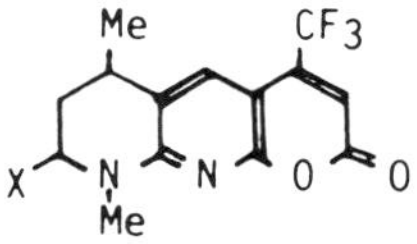

#M379 X=H; #M380 X=Me

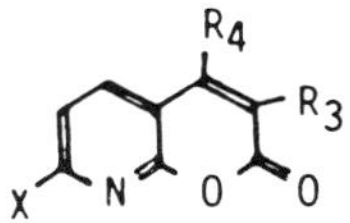

#M375- #M378

Dye no.	R_3	R_4	R_5	R_6	R_7	R_8
#M277	H	Me	OH	CH_3CO	H	H
#M278	H	H	H	H	OH	H
#M279	CN	H	H	H	OH	H
#M280	C_2H_5COO	H	H	H	OH	H

(continued)

233

Table 23 (continued)

Dye no.	R_3	R_4	R_5	R_6	R_7	R_8
#M281	H	Me	H	H	OH	H
#M282	H	CF_3	H	H	OH	H
#M283	CN	Me	H	H	OH	H
#M284	Ph	Me	H	H	OH	H
#M285	isopropyl	Me	H	H	OH	H
#M286	Et	Me	H	H	OH	H
#M287	$n-C_4H_9$	Me	H	H	OH	H
#M288	CH_2-Ph	Me	H	H	OH	H
#M290	H	Me	H	H	OH	Me
#M291	H	H	H	H	OH	(1)
#M292	H	Me	H	H	OH	(1)
#M293	H	H	H	CH_3O	OH	H
#M294	H	H	H	(2)	OH	H
#M295	H	Me	OH	H	OH	H

234

#M296	H	Me	H	OH	OH	H
#M297	Biphenyl	H	H	H	OMe	H
#M298	(3)	H	H	H	OMe	H
#M299	(4)	H	H	H	OMe	H
#M300	C_2H_5COO	H	H	H	OMe	H
#M301	H	Me	H	H	OCOMe	H
#M302	Ph	H	H	H	OCOMe	H
#M303	H	Me	Allyl	H	OCOMe	Me
#M304	(5)	Me	H	H	OCOMe	H
#M305	H	Me	H	Allyl	OCOMe	Me
#M306	Ph	H	H	H	OCOMe	H
#M307	Ph	Amyl	H	H	OCOMe	H
#M315	H	Me	H	Me	NHMe	H
#M320	H	Me	H	Me	NHEt	H
#M321	H	CF_3	H	Me	NHEt	H

(continued)

235

Table 23 *(continued)*

Dye no.	X	R_3	R_4
#M308	(6)	H	Me
#M309	NH_2	H	H
#M310	NH_2	Ph	H
#M311	NH_2	H	Me
#M312	NH_2	H	CF_3
#M313	NH_2	H	OMe
#M314	NH_2	Et	Me
#M316	$NHCH_2SO_3Na$	H	Me
#M317	$NHCH_2SO_3Na$	Ph	H
#M318	$NHCH_2CH_2OH$	H	Me
#M319	NHEt	H	CF_3
#M322	$NH(CH_2)_3SO_3Na$	H	Me
#M323	$NH(CH_2)_4SO_3Na$	H	Me
#M324	NMe_2	H	H

Dye no.	X	R_3	R_4
#M325	NMe_2	C_2H_5COO	H
#M326	NMe_2	H	Me_2
#M327	NMe_2	H	CF_3
#M328	NMe_2	Me	OH
#M329	NEt_2	H	H
#M330	NEt_2	H	Me
#M331	NEt_2	Et	Me
#M332	NEt_2	(7)	H
#M333	NEt_2	H	CF_3
#M334	NEt_2	(8)	H
#M335	NEt_2	(9)	H
#M336	NEt_2	(10)	H
#M337	NEt_2	(11)	H
#M338	$NMe(CH_2)_4SO_3Na$	H	Me

#			
#M339	Me	H	N[(CH$_2$)$_3$SO$_3$Na]$_2$
#M340	Me	H	N[(CH$_2$)$_4$SO$_3$Na]$_2$
#M341	H	Ph	(12)
#M342	H	H	H
#M343	H	H	Me
#M344	CF$_3$	H	H
#M345	CF$_3$	H	Me
#M346	CF$_3$	H	Et
#M347	Me	H	(CH$_2$)$_3$SO$_3$Na
#M348	Me	H	(CH$_2$)$_4$SO$_3$Na
#M349	CF$_3$	H	H
#M350	CF$_3$	H	Me
#M351	H	H	—
#M352	Me	H	—
#M353	CF$_3$	H	—
#M355	H	COMe	—
#M356	H	CN	—

#			
#M357	—	COOH	H
#M358	—	C$_2$H$_5$COO	H
#M359	—	CH$_2$COOH	H
#M360	(13)-Ph	Ph	H
#M361	(14)-PhMe	Ph	H
#M362	(14)-MeEt	(15)	H
#M363	(14)-PhMe	(15)	H
#M364	(16)	p-tolyl	H
#M365	(15)	p-tolyl	H
#M366	(15)-Me$_2$	Ph-OCH$_3$	H
#M367	(13)-MeCl	(17)	H
#M368	(18)	(13)-Cl	H
#M369	(14)-MeEt	(17)	H
#M370	(17)	p-tolyl	H
#M375	OH	H	Me
#M376	NH$_2$	Me	Me
#M377	NMe$_2$	H	Me
#M378	(19)	H	Me

Table 24. Abbreviations Used in Table 23

(1) $-CH_2N\begin{smallmatrix}CH_2COOH\\CH_2COOH\end{smallmatrix}$

(2) (sugar/glucose structure with OH, H, CH_2OH, O)

(3) $-N^+(CH_3)_3 \quad CH_3SO_4^-$ (benzene ring)

(4) $-N\!=\!\overset{+}{N}-CH_3 \quad CH_3SO_4^-$

(5) (tetrahydronaphthalene structure)

(6) $-CO_2-CH_2-CH_2-CH_3$

(7) (benzimidazolium) Me–N$^+$–N–Me $\quad Cl^-$

(8) (benzothiazole) S, N

(9) (chlorobenzothiazole) S, N, Cl

(10) (benzimidazole) H–N, N

(11) (N-methyl benzimidazole) Me–N, N

(12) Et Et N–C, N / Cl^- C–N, C–NH–

(13) (pyrazole) –N, N

(14) (imidazole/triazole) –N, N

(15) –N, N

(16) –N, N

(17) –N, $\overset{+}{N}-CH_3 \quad CH_3SO_4^-$

(18) Me (benzimidazolium) $\overset{+}{N}$, N $\quad OC_4H_9$

(19) (morpholine) –N, O

238

Table 25. Laser Characteristics of Quinolone and Azaquinolone Derivatives[a]

Solvent	Concentration (mM)	Lasing wavelength (tuning) (nm)	Excitation	Output	Ref.
#M381	2,7-Dihydroxy-4-methylquinoline; 7-Hydroxy-4-methylquinolone-2				
Ethanol + NaOH	2	423–463 (grating)	N$_2$ (530 kW, 3.5 ns)	E = 6.9%	139
Ethanol + NaOH		441 (BB)	Fl (200 ns, RT)	Thr = 24 J	184
#M382	7-Hydroxy-3,4-dimethylquinolone-2				
Ethanol + NaOH		447	Fl (200 ns, RT)	Thr = 20 J	184
#M383	7-Amino quinolone-2				
Ethanol		418 (BB)	Fl (200 ns, RT)	Thr = 24 J	184
#M384	2-Hydroxy-4-methyl-7-aminoquinoline; 7-amino-4-methylquinolone-2; carbostyril 124				
Ethanol		413 (BB)	Fl (1.2 μs, RT)		225

(continued)

Table 25 (*continued*)

Solvent	Concentration (mM)	Lasing wavelength (tuning) (nm)	Excitation	Output	Ref.
Ethanol		413 (BB)	Fl (200 ns, RT)	Thr = 18 J	184
#M385 7-Amino-4-trifluoromethylquinolone-2; Q1F					
Ethanol	0.75	463 (BB)	Fl (5 J)	4 kW	222
#M386 7-Dimethylamino-4-methylquinolone-2; carbostyril 165					
Ethanol		425 (BB)	Fl (1.2 µs, RT)		225
EG	3	414–490 (BF filter)	Ar (351 and 364 nm, 1.5 W)	70 mW	35
Methanol	0.2	430–440 (grating)	Fl (86 J)	10 mJ	100
Ethanol	0.3	425 (BB)	Fl (100 J, 150 ns, RT)	150 mJ	186
#M387 7-Diethylamino-4-methylquinolone-2					
Ethanol		425 (BB)	Fl (200 ns, RT)	Thr = 16 J	184

#	Compound	Solvent				
#M388	7-Amino-1-methylquinolone-2	Ethanol	412 (BB)	Fl (200 ns, RT)	Thr = 20 J	184
#M389	7-Amino-1,4-dimethylquinolone-2	Ethanol	409 (BB)	Fl (200 ns, RT)	Thr = 20 J	184
#M390	7-Amino-4,8-dimethylquinolone-2	Ethanol	420 (BB)	Fl (200 ns, RT)	Thr = 26 J	184
#M391	7-Dimethylamino-1-methylquinolone-2	Ethanol	(BB)	Fl (200 ns, RT)	Thr = 24 J	184
#M392	7-Dimethylamino-1,4-dimethylquinolone-2	Ethanol	420 (BB)	Fl (200 ns, RT)	Thr = 12 J	184
#M393	7-Dimethylamino-1-methyl-4-trifluoromethylquinolone-2; Q3F	Ethanol	0.75	477 (BB)	Fl (5 J)	5 kW; Q3F	222
#M394	7-Dimethylamino-1-methyl-4-methoxyquinolone-2	Ethanol + NaOH	409 (BB)	Fl (200 ns, RT)	Thr = 40 J	184

(continued)

Table 25 (continued)

Solvent	Concentration (mM)	Lasing wavelength (tuning) (nm)	Excitation	Output	Ref.
#M395 5-Dimethylamino-1-methylquinolone-2					
Ethanol	5	(BB)	N$_2$ (20 kW, 10 ns)		184
#M396 4-Methyl-2(1H)-pyrrolidino[4,5-g]quinolone; compound 857-11-c5					
Ethanol		422 (BB)	Fl (200 ns, RT)	Thr = 18 J	184
#M397 4,6,6,7-Tetramethyl-2(1H)-pyrrolidino[4,5-g]quinolone; LD 423; violet 2; compound 857-109					
Ethanol		423 (BB)	Fl (200 ns, RT)	Thr = 20 J	184
Methanol	0.2	415–447 (grating)	Fl (150 ns, RT, 1 Hz)		87
#M398 6,6,7,8-Tetramethyl-4-trifluoromethyl-2(1H)-pyrrolidino[4,5-g]quinolone; Q4F					
Ethanol	0.75	477 (BB)	Fl (5 J)	4 kW	222

#M399 1,6,6,7,8-Pentamethyl-4-trifluoromethyl-2(1H)-pyrrolidino[4,5-g]quinolone; LD 473; blue 5; Q6F

Solvent					
Ethanol	0.75	473 (BB)	Fl (5 J)	10 kW	222
Methanol	0.08	454-522 (grating)	Fl (150 ns, RT, 1 Hz)		87

#M400 7-Hydroxy-4-methyl-8-azaquinolone-2

Ethanol		395 (BB)	Fl (200 ns, RT)	Thr = 22 J	184

#M401 7-Hydroxy-3,4-dimethyl-8-azaquinolone-2

Ethanol		405 (BB)	Fl (200 ns, RT)	Thr = 40 J	184

#M402 7-Amino-8-azaquinolone-2

Ethanol	5	(BB)	N_2 (20 kW, 10 ns)		184

#M403 7-Amino-4-trifluoromethyl-8-azaquinolone-2

Ethanol		437 (BB)	Fl (200 ns, RT)	Thr = 28 J	184

#M404 7-Amino-4-methoxy-8-azaquinolone-2

Ethanol	5	(BB)	N_2 (20 kW, 10 ns)		184

(continued)

Table 25 *(continued)*

Solvent	Concentration (mM)	Lasing wavelength (tuning) (nm)	Excitation	Output	Ref.
#M405 7-Amino-4-methyl-8-azaquinolone-2					
Ethanol		386 (BB)	Fl (200 ns, RT)	Thr = 40 J	184
#M406 7-Dimethylamino-1,4-dimethyl-8-azaquinolone-2					
Ethanol		407 (BB)	Fl (200 ns, RT)	Thr = 14 J	184
iso-Propanol + 10% water		405 (BB)	Fl (200 ns, RT)	Thr = 9 J	
			Fl (70 J, 400–600 ns, RT)	Thr = 30 J	
#M407 7-Dimethylamino-1-methyl-4-trifluoromethyl-8-azaquinolone-2; AQ1F					
Ethanol	0.75	452 (BB)	Fl (5 J)	6 kW	222
#M408 7-Dimethylamino-1-methyl-4-methoxy-8-azaquinolone-2; LD 390					
Ethanol		390 (BB)	Fl (200 ns, RT)	Thr = 20 J	184
			Fl (70 J, 400–600 ns, RT)	Thr = 48 J	

#M409 1-Methyl-4-trifluoromethyl-7-methoxy-8-azaquinolone-2

Ethanol	5	(BB)	N_2 (20 kW, 10 ns)	184

#M410 5,8-Dimethyl-5,6,7,8-tetrahydro-8-azaquinolone-2

		(Grating)	N_2 (20 kW, 10 ns)	184

[a]Chemical structures of quinolone and azaquinolone derivatives.

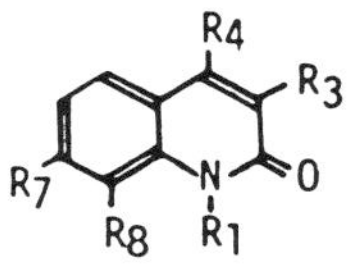

#M381- #M394

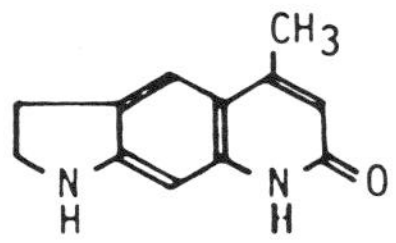

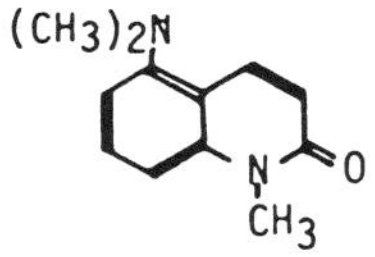

#M395

#M396

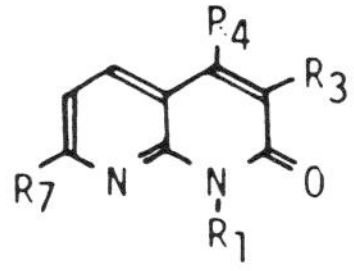

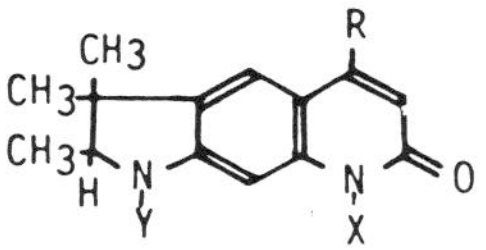

#M397 X=H, Y=H, R=Me

#M398 X=H, Y=Me, R=CF₃

#M399 X=Me, Y=Me, R=CF₃

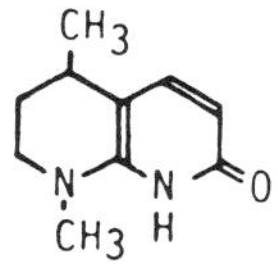

#M400- #M409

#M410

(continued)

245

Table 25 (continued)

Dye no.	R_1	R_3	R_4	R_7	R_8
#M381	H	H	Me	OH	H
#M382	H	Me	Me	OH	H
#M383	H	H	H	NH_2	H
#M384	H	H	Me	NH_2	H
#M385	H	H	CF_3	NH_2	H
#M386	H	H	Me	NMe_2	H
#M387	H	H	Me	NEt_2	H
#M388	Me	H	H	NH_2	H
#M389	Me	H	Me	NH_2	H
#M390	H	H	Me	NH_2	Me
#M391	Me	H	H	NMe_2	H
#M392	Me	H	Me	NMe_2	H

Dye no.	R_1	R_3	R_4	R_7	R_8
#M393	Me	H	CF_3	NMe_2	H
#M394	Me	H	OCH_3	NMe_2	H
#M400	H	H	Me	OH	—
#M401	H	Me	Me	OH	—
#M402	H	H	H	NH_2	—
#M403	H	H	CF_3	NH_2	—
#M404	H	H	OCH_3	NH_2	—
#M405	H	H	Me	NH_2	—
#M406	Me	H	Me	NMe_2	—
#M407	Me	H	CF_3	NMe_2	—
#M408	Me	H	OCH_3	NMe_2	—
#M409	Me	H	CF_3	OCH_3	—

Table 26. Laser Characteristics of Oxazole and Benzoxazole Derivatives[a]

Solvent	Concentration (mM)	Lasing wavelength (tuning) (nm)	Excitation	Output	Ref.
#M411 2,5-Diphenyloxazole; PPO					
Toluene	0.7-10	358.3-390.5 (BB, concentration + solvent)	N_2 (20-40 kW, 10 Hz)	E = 1%	232
Benzene	2-5				
Dioxane	0.2-2				
Dioxane	7	381 (BB)	Fl (20 J, 50 ns, RT)	Thr = 17 J	137
Cyclohexane	1	357 (BB)	N_2 (200 kW, 3 ns, 10 Hz)	1.4 kW	71
Toluene	6	359-391 (grating)	N_2 (270 kW)	23 kW	220
Cyclohexane	1	372 (BB)	KrF (0.2 J, 20 ns)	E = 2.5%	120
Cyclohexane	5	370-380 (tuned)	KrF	E = 10%	182

(continued)

Table 26 (continued)

Solvent	Concentration (mM)	Lasing wavelength (tuning) (nm)	Excitation	Output	Ref.
Ethanol	1	378 (BB)	XeCl (60 mJ, 35 ns)	E = 2.3%	95
Cyclohexane	5	354–361 and 368–382 (grating) (osc + amp)	YAG–FH (5 mJ, 5 ns, 10 Hz)	E = 1.6%	183
#M412 2-Phenyl-5-(4-difluoromethylsulfonylphenyl) oxazole					
Toluene	1	405–430 (grating)	N_2 (600 kW, 5 ns, 5–50 Hz)	55 kW	200
#M413 2-(4-Pyridyl)-5-phenyloxazole; 4PyPO					
Ethanol	1	395–402 (grating)	N_2 (100 kW, 10 ns, 100 Hz)		243
#M414 4-{2-(5-Phenyloxazolyl)} pyridinium hydrochloride; 4PyPO–HCl					
Water (pH = 2)	1	504 (BB)	N_2 (100 kW, 10 ns, 100 Hz)		243

Solvent	Conc	Wavelength	Pump	Output	Ref
Water (pH = 2)		504 (BB)	Fl (5 J)	4.8 kW	

#M415 4-{2-(5-Phenyloxazolyl)}-1-methylphridinium p-toluenesulfonate; 4PyPO-MePTS

Solvent	Conc	Wavelength	Pump	Output	Ref
Water	1	470–549 (grating)	N_2 (100 kW, 10 ns, 100 Hz)		243
Water		506	Fl (5 J)	2.3 kW	

#M416 2-(1-Naphthyl)-5-phenyloxazole; α NPO

Solvent	Conc	Wavelength	Pump	Output	Ref
Toluene	3.7	399.5 (BB)	Nd-TH (8 MW)	E = 6.5%	177
Ethanol	1	397.5 (BB)	Ruby-SH (0.8 MW, 12 ns)	80 kW	193
Cyclohexane	1	393 (BB)			
Benzene	1	402 (BB)			
Ethanol, toluene, benzene, or cyclohexane	10	392–413.5 (BB, solvent)	N_2 (20–40 kW, 10 Hz)	E = 3%	232
Ethanol	0.25	400 (BB)	Fl (20 J, 50 ns, RT)	Thr = 10 J	137

(continued)

Table 26 (continued)

Solvent	Concentration (mM)	Lasing wavelength (tuning) (nm)	Excitation	Output	Ref.
Cyclohexane	0.5	392.6 (BB)	N_2 (200 kW, 3 ns, 10 Hz)	4 kW	71
		390–395 (grating)	N_2 (120 kW, 10 ns, 100 Hz)	E = 12% (8 ns)	130
Toluene	2.5	393–426 (grating)	N_2 (270 kW)	40 kW	220
Dioxane	1	401 (BB)	Fl (9 J, 80 ns)	Thr = 4.2 J	1
Cyclohexane	0.3	398 (BB)	Ruby-SH (8 MW, 8 ns)	0.9 MW	73
Vapor		(BB)	N_2 (1 MW)		245

#M417 2-Phenyl-5-(4-biphenyl) oxazole; PBO

Solvent	Concentration (mM)	Lasing wavelength (tuning) (nm)	Excitation	Output	Ref.
Dioxane	2	383–386 and 402–409 (grating)	N_2 (530 kW, 3.5 ns)	E = 17.8%	139
Ethanol	1	388.5 (BB)	XeCl (60 mJ, 35 ns)	E = 7.8%	95

#M418 2-(4-Biphenylyl)-5-phenyloxazole; BPO

Vapor		368–394 (grating)	N_2 (1 MW, 4.5 ns)		244

#M419 2,5-Bis(4-biphenylyl) oxazole; BBO

Toluene	2.6	409 (BB)	Nd–TH (8 MW)	E = 4%	177
Benzene	1	408.5 (BB)	Ruby–SH (0.8 MW, 12 ns)		193
Toluene	0.1–1	401–419.5 (BB, concentration)	N_2 (20–40 kW, 10 Hz)	E = 14%	232
DMF	0.3	413.7 (BB)	N_2 (200 kW, 3 ns, 10 Hz)	14.2 kW	71
Benzene	Satur. ×0.05	410 (BB)	Fl (20 J, 50 ns, RT)	Thr = 10.2 J	173
Benzene	1	400–419 (grating)	N_2 (100 kW, 10 ns, 100 Hz)		185
Dioxane	1	410 (BB)	Fl (9 J, 80 ns, RT)	Thr = 3.3 J	1
Vapor		(BB)	N_2 (1 MW)		245

#M420 2-(4-Biphenylyl)-5-(1-naphthyl) oxazole

Toluene	0.01–1	413 (BB)	Nd–TH (0.04 J, 40 ns)		168
PMMA		410 (BB)			

(continued)

Table 26 (continued)

Solvent	Concentration (mM)	Lasing wavelength (tuning) (nm)	Excitation	Output	Ref.
#M421 5-Phenyl-2-(p-styrylphenyl) oxazole					
Toluene	0.01-1	417 (BB)	Nd-TH (0.04 J, 40 ns)		168
PMMA		414 (BB)			
#M422 5-Phenyl-2-[p-(p-phenylstyryl)phenyl] oxazole					
Toluene	0.01-1	432 (BB)	Nd-TH (0.04 J, 40 ns)		168
PMMA		428 (BB)			
#M423 2-[p-[2-(2-Naphthyl)vinyl]phenyl]-5-phenyloxazole					
Toluene	0.01-1	428 (BB)	Nd-TH (0.04 J, 40 ns)		168
PMMA		425 (BB)			
#M424 2-[p-[2-(9-Anthryl)vinyl]phenyl]-5-phenyloxazole					
PMMA	0.01-1	480 (BB)	Nd-TH (0.04 J, 40 ns)		168

252

(continued)

#M425 5-(4-Biphenylyl)-2-[p-(4-phenyl-1,3-butadienyl)phenyl] oxazole

Solvent	Conc.	Wavelength (nm)	Pump	Output	Ref.
Toluene	0.01–1	448 (BB)	Nd–TH (0.04 J, 40 ns)		168
PMMA		443 (BB)			

#M426 p-Bis(5-phenyloxazolyl) benzene; POPOP

Solvent	Conc.	Wavelength (nm)	Pump	Output	Ref.
Toluene		417 (BB)	Nd–TH (1 MW)		76
Ethanol	1	421 (BB)	Ruby–SH (0.8 MW, 12 ns)		193
Toluene	0.34	419 (BB)	Fl (90 J, 100 ns, RT)	12 kW (Thr = 42 J)	138
Benzene, toluene, cyclohexane or dioxane	0.01–10	412–431 (BB, concentration + solvent)	N_2 (20–40 kW, 10 Hz)	E = 20%	232
		390–445 (grating)	N_2 (120 kW, 10 ns, 100 Hz)	E = 18% (8 ns)	130
Ethanol	1	420–446 (grating)	Ruby–SH (5 MW, 15 ns)	40 kW	79
Xylene	1	415.8–428.1, 435.6–441.3 (grating)	N_2 (100 kW)		194

Table 26 *(continued)*

Solvent	Concentration (mM)	Lasing wavelength (tuning) (nm)	Excitation	Output	Ref.
Toluene	0.5	419 (BB)	Fl (9 J, 80 ns)	Thr = 2.9 J	1
Tetra-hydrofuran	5	409–430 (prism + grating)	N_2 (130 kW)	13.7 kW	13
Dioxane	1	407–451.5 (grating)	N_2 (270 kW)	80 kW	220
Vapor	(410°C)	399.3 (BB)	N_2 (0.9 MW)	1 kW	246
Vapor	(330°C)	393 (BB)	N_2 (400 kW, 10 ns)	30 kW, Thr = 50 kW	247
Vapor + Ar + N_2	5 Torr: 2 atm: 4 atm	381 (BB)	REB (1 MeV, 28 kA, 30 ns)	500 kW (10 ns)	248
Dioxane	2	419 (BB)	XeCl (60 mJ, 35 ns)	E = 20.2%	95

#M427 1,4-Bis(4-methyl-5-phenyloxazolyl)benzene; dimethyl POPOP

Solvent	Conc.	Wavelength	Pump		Ref.
Cyclohexane	1	423 (BB)	Ruby-SH (0.8 MW, 12 ns)		193
Ethanol	1	431 (BB)			
Benzene, toluene, or cyclohexane	0.05–5	423.5–441 (BB, concentration + solvent)	N_2 (20–40 kW, 10 Hz)	E = 16%	232
Toluene	0.01–1	425 (BB)	Nd-TH (0.04 J, 40 ns)		168
Toluene	0.5	431 (BB)	Fl (9 J, 80 ns, RT)	Thr = 4.2 J	1
Dioxane	0.7	418–465 (grating)	N_2 (270 kW)	80 kW	220
Vapor		410 (BB)	N_2 (400 kW, 10 ns)	Thr = 200 kW	247
Cyclohexane	0.3	431 (BB)	Ruby-SH (8 MW, 8 ns)	0.6 MW	73
Ethanol	0.1	420 (BB)	Fl (100 J, 150 ns, RT)		186
Dioxane	0.7	432 (grating)	YAG-TH (10.5 MW, 8 ns, 20 Hz)	250 mWav.	221

#M428 1,4-Bis[2-(4-butoxy-5-phenyloxazolyl)]benzene; dibutoxy POPOP

Solvent	Conc.	Wavelength	Pump		Ref.
Ethanol		448–454 (BB)	Fl (50 J, 200 ns, RT)	Thr = 35 J	249

(continued)

Table 26 (continued)

Solvent	Concentration (mM)	Lasing wavelength (tuning) (nm)	Excitation	Output	Ref.
#M429 Methyl-p-terphenylmethyl POPOP; TP-C-DMP					
Dioxane	0.1	(BB)	Fl (145 J)	35 kW (130 ns)	257
#M430 1,4-Bis[5-(4-biphenylyl)-2-oxazolyl]benzene; BOPOB					
Tetra-hydrofuran		428-450 (grating)	N_2 (100 kW)		185
Vapor		359-393 (grating)	N_2 (1 MW, 4.5 ns)		244
#M431 1,4-Bis[5-(1-naphthylyl)-2-oxazolyl]benzene; α NOPON					
		430-445 (grating)	N_2 (120 kW, 10 ns, 100 Hz)	E = 18% (6 ns)	130
Benzene		430-455 (grating)	N_2 (100 kW)		185

#M432 1,4-Bis[2-(5-*p*-tolyloxazol)]benzene; TOPOT

Vapor	(623 K)	380–425 (grating)	N_2 (1 MW, 4.5 ns)		244

#M433 1,4-Bis{4-[5-(4-biphenylyl)-2-oxazolyl]styryl}benzene

Toluene	0.01–1	460 (BB)	Nd–TH (0.04 J, 40 ns)		168
PMMA		455 (BB)			

#M434 1,2-Bis(5-phenyloxazolyl)ethylene

Toluene	0.01–1	447 (BB)	Nd–TH (0.04 J, 40 ns)		168
PMMA		444 (BB)			

#M435 2-Phenylbenzoxazole

Cyclohexane		330 and 345 (BB)	Nd–FH (25 ps, 0.12 mJ) (2.5 ns, 40 mJ)	E = 20%	250

#M436 1,2-Bis(5-methyl-2-benzoxazolyl)ethylene

Dichloromethane 1		425 (BB)	N_2 (1 MW, 2.5 ns)		155
Vapor			N_2 (1 MW)		245

(continued)

Table 26 (continued)

Solvent	Concentration (mM)	Lasing wavelength (tuning) (nm)	Excitation	Output	Ref.
#M437 2,5-Bis[5-tert-butyl-2-benzoxazolyl]thiophene; BBOT					
Benzene	0.5	437 (BB)	Fl (20 J, 50 ns, RT)	Thr = 7.4 J	137
Xylene	5	429.4-442.4 (grating)	N_2 (100 kW)		194
Dioxane	1	433 (BB)	Fl (9 J, 80 ns, RT)	Thr = 6.2 J	1
Dioxane	2	431-436 and 455-463 (grating)	N_2 (530 kW, 3.5 ns)	E = 15.5%	139
#M438 2-(4-Biphenylyl)-5-phenylbenzoxazole; PBBO					
Toluene + ethanol (7:3)	0.5	391-411 (grating) (osc + amp)	N_2 (1 MW, 10 ns, 50 Hz)	0.5 mJ	97

a Chemical structures of oxazole and benzoxazole derivatives. The symbols (a)-(i) are shown in Table 27.

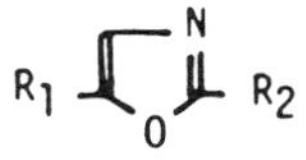

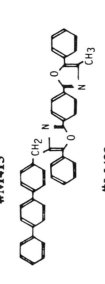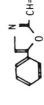

#M411- #M414 ; #M416- #M420

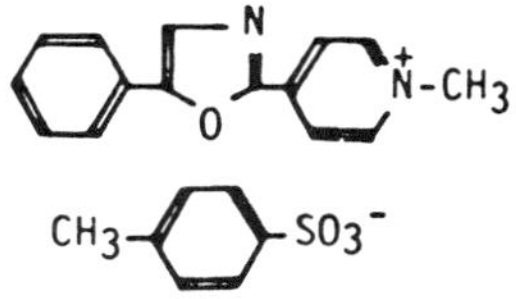

#M415

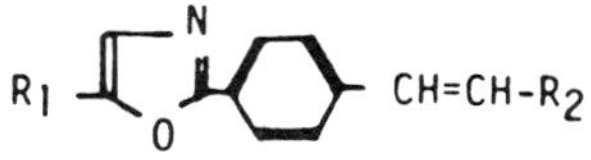

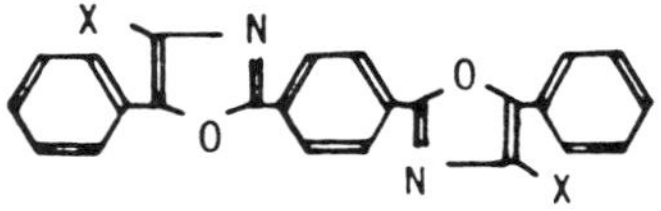

#M426 X=H ; #M427 X=Me ;
#M428 X=OC₄H₉,
(estimated)

#M429

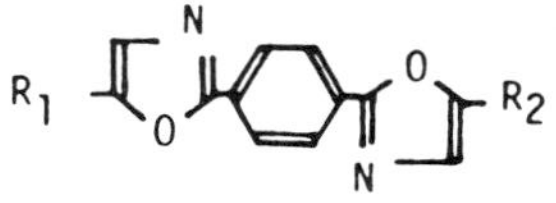

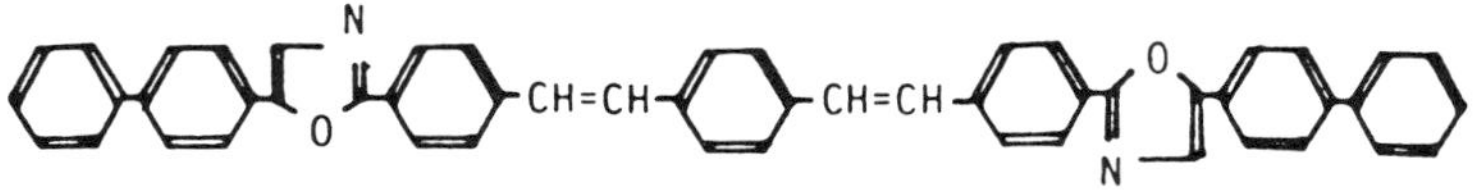

#M433

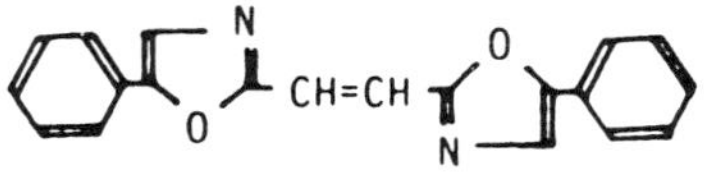

#M434

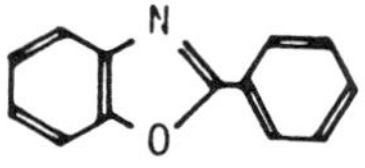

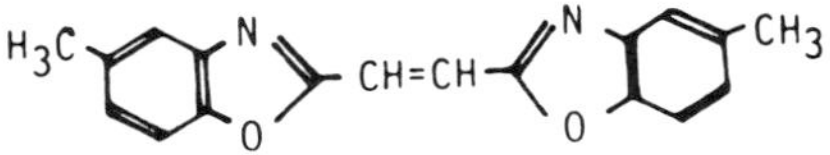

#M436

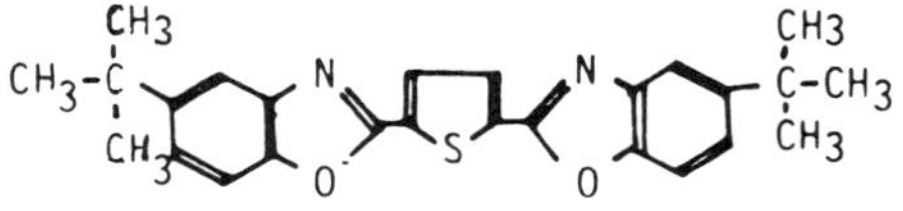

#M437

#M421- #M425

#M430- #M432

#M435

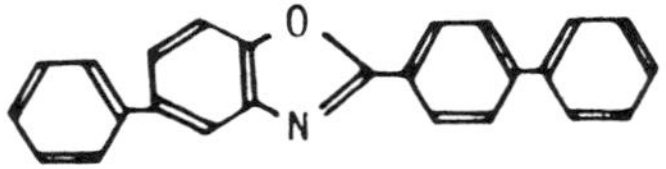

#M438

(continued)

259

Table 26 (continued)

Dye no.	R$_1$	R$_2$	Dye no.	R$_1$	R$_2$
#M411	Ph	Ph	#M420	(c)	(d)
#M412	(a); X = SO$_2$CHF$_2$	Ph	#M421	Ph	Ph
#M413	Ph	(b)	#M422	Ph	(d)
#M414	Ph	(b); HCl	#M423	Ph	(e)
#M416	Ph	(c)	#M424	Ph	(f)
#M417	Ph	(d)	#M425	(d)	(g)
#M418	(d)	Ph	#M430	(d)	(d)
#M419	(d)	(d)	#M431	(c)	(c)
			#M432	(a); X = Me	(a); X = Me

Table 27. Abbreviations Used in Table 26

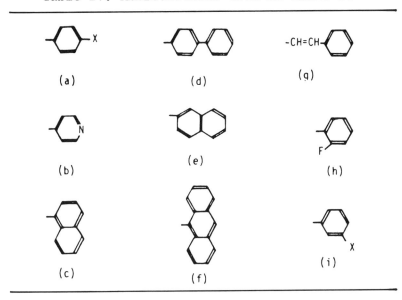

(a)

(b)

(c)

(d)

(e)

(f)

(g)

(h)

(i)

Table 28. Laser Characteristics of Oxadiazole Derivatives[a]

Solvent	Concentration (mM)	Lasing wavelength (tuning) (nm)	Excitation	Output	Ref.
#M439 2,5-Diphenyl-1,3,4-oxadiazole; PPD					
Ethanol	1	347 (BB)	Nd–FH (600 kW)	Thr = 50 kW	178
Dioxane	9	348 (BB)	Fl (20 J, 50 ns, RT)	Thr = 20 J	137
Ethanol	>1	383–395 (grating)	N_2 (100 kW)		185
Cyclohexane	10	348 (BB)	CO_2-laser-produced plasma (10 J)	0.3 mJ	187
		350 (BB)	Glass–FH (6 ps, 1–3 mJ, single pulse)	10 µJ, E = 1% (ps pulse)	93
#M440 2-(2-Fluorophenyl)-5-phenyl-1,3,4-oxadiazole					
Ethanol	5	347.4 (BB)	KrF (6 mJ, 5 ns)	E = 12%	251
#M441 2-(3-Fluorophenyl)-5-phenyl-1,3,4-oxadiazole					
Cyclohexane	5	346.6 (BB)	KrF (6 mJ, 5 ns)	E = 3%	251

Solvent	Conc.	Compound	λ (BB)	Pump	Efficiency	Ref.
Ethanol	5	#M442 2-(4-Fluorophenyl)-5-phenyl-1,3,4-oxadiazole	347.2 (BB)	KrF (6 mJ, 5 ns)	E = 11%	251
Ethanol	5	#M443 2-(4-Bromophenyl)-5-phenyl-1,3,4-oxadiazole	352.9 (BB)	KrF (6 mJ, 5 ns)	E = 1.5%	251
Ethanol	5	#M444 2-(2,4-Dichlorophenyl)-5-phenyl-1,3,4-oxadiazole	358.5 (BB)	KrF (6 mJ, 5 ns)	E = 2%	251
Ethanol	5	#M445 2-(3,4-Dichlorophenyl)-5-phenyl-1,3,4-oxadiazole	356.8 (BB)	KrF (6 mJ, 5 ns)	E = 5%	251
Ethanol	1.1	#M446 2-Phenyl-5-(p-methoxyphenyl)-1,3,4-oxadiazole	365 (BB)	Nd-FH (600 kW)	Thr = 80 kW	178
Toluene	0.01–1	#M447 2-(p-Dimethylaminophenyl)-5-phenyl-1,3,4-oxadiazole	408 (BB)	Nd-TH (0.04 J, 40 ns)		168
Ethanol	5	#M448 2,5-Bis(2-fluorophenyl)-1,3,4-oxadiazole	346.5 (BB)	KrF (6 mJ, 5 ns)	E = 9%	251

(continued)

Table 28 (continued)

Solvent	Concentration (mM)	Lasing wavelength (tuning) (nm)	Excitation	Output	Ref.
#M449 2,5-Bis(3-flurophenyl)-1,3,4-oxadiazole					
Ethanol	5	347 (BB)	KrF (6 mJ, 5 ns)	E = 9%	251
#M450 2,5-Bis(4-chlorophenyl)-1,3,4-oxadiazole					
Ethanol	5	357 (BB)	KrF (6 mJ, 5 ns)	E = 10%	251
#M451 2,5-Bis(p-methoxyphenyl)-1,3,4-oxadiazole					
Ethanol	1	359 and 372 (BB)	Nd-FH (600 kW)	Thr = 80 kW	178
#M452 2,5-Bis(p-diethylaminophenyl)-1,3,4-oxadiazole					
Dichloro-methane	1	425 (BB)	N$_2$ (1 MW, 2.5 ns)		155
#M453 2-(p-Chlorophenyl)-5-(p-dimethylaminophenyl)-1,3,4-oxadiazole					
Toluene	0.01-1	420 (BB)	Nd-TH (0.04 J, 40 ns)		168

#M454 2-Phenyl-5-[p-(4-phenyl-1,3-butadienyl)phenyl]-1,3,4-oxadiazole

Toluene	0.01–1	424 (BB)	Nd-TH (0.04 J, 40 ns)		168
PMMA		418 (BB)			

#M455 2-Phenyl-5-(4-biphenylyl)-1,3,4-oxadiazole; PBD

Toluene	0.4–40	377–415 (BB, concentration)	N_2 (20–40 kW, 10 Hz)		232
Ethanol		355–382 (grating)	N_2 (100 kW)		185
Ethanol	Satur. ×0.1	362.5 (BB)	Fl (20 J, 50 ns, RT)	Thr = 5.4 J	137
Dioxane	1	360 (BB)	Fl (9 J, 80 ns, RT)	Thr = 4.2 J	1
Toluene	5	357–376 (grating)	N_2 (530 kW, 3.5 ns)	E = 19.2%	139
Toluene	7	357–388 (grating)	N_2 (270 kW)	72 kW	220
Cyclohexane	5	355 (BB)	KrF (0.2 J, 20 ns)	E = 15%	120
Ethanol	0.5	362.5 (BB)	XeCl (60 mJ, 35 ns)	E = 13.9%	95

(continued)

265

Table 28 (continued)

Solvent	Concentration (mM)	Lasing wavelength (tuning) (nm)	Excitation	Output	Ref.
Toluene + ethanol (1:1)		360–386 (grating) (osc + amp)	N_2 (1 MW, 10 ns, 50 Hz)	0.3 mJ	97
Cyclohexane	0.37	351–385 (grating) (osc + amp)	KrF or XeCl (150–250 mJ, 10–20 ns)	E = 4%	26
#M456 2-(4-tert-Butylphenyl)-5-(4-biphenylyl)-1,3,4-oxadiazole; butyl PBD; U.V. 2; BPBD					
Toluene	2	362–367 and 373–392 (grating)	N_2 (530 kW, 3.5 ns)	E = 17%	139
Toluene	4	357–395 (grating)	N_2 (270 kW)	85 kW	220
Ethanol		361–371 (grating + prism) (osc + amp)	KrF (1 MW, 7 ns, 20–50 Hz)		252

Solvent	Conc.	Wavelength	Laser	Efficiency	Ref.
Cyclohexane	5	354–388 (grating) (osc + amp)	YAG–FH (5 mJ, 5 ns, 10 Hz)	E = 4.7%	183
Cyclohexane	0.6	351–385 (grating) (osc + amp)	KrF or XeCl (150–250 mJ, 10–20 ns)	E = 8%	26
Hexane	0.46	354–385 (grating) (osc + amp)		E = 9%	
DMF	0.2	355–380 (grating)	Fl (150 ns, RT, 1 Hz)		87

#M457 2-(4-isopropylphenyl)-5-(4-biphenylyl)-1,3,4-oxadiazole; isopropyl PBD

Ethanol	0.8	369.8 (BB)	Fl (20 J, 50 ns, RT)	Thr = 4.8 J	137
Cyclohexane	0.8	361 (BB)		Thr = 6 J	
Toluene	11	363–385 (grating)	N_2 (100 kW)		194

#M458 2-(4-Biphenylyl)-5-(p-styrylphenyl)-1,3,4-oxadiazole

Toluene	0.01–1	403 (BB)	Nd–TH 0.04 J, 40 ns)		168
PMMA		400 (BB)			

(continued)

Table 28 *(continued)*

Solvent	Concentration (mM)	Lasing wavelength (tuning) (nm)	Excitation	Output	Ref.
	#M459 2-(1-Naphthyl)-5-phenyl-1,3,4-oxadiazole; αNPD				
Benzene	5	373 and 391 (BB)	Ruby-SH (5 MW, 20 ns)	2.5 MW	164
	#M460 2-(1-Naphthyl)-5-(4-methoxyphenyl)-1,3,4-oxadiazole; 4-methoxy-αNPD				
Toluene	3	379 (BB)	N_2 (3 ns)		253
	#M461 2-(1-Naphthyl)-5-(4-bromophenyl)-1,3,4-oxadiazole; 4-bromo-αNPD				
Toluene	3	376.5 (BB)	N_2 (3 ns)		253
	#M462 2-(1-Naphthyl)-5-(2-fluorophenyl)-1,3,4-oxadiazole; 2-fluoro-αNPD				
Toluene	4.5	373 (BB)	N_2 (3 ns)		253
	#M463 2-(1-Naphthyl)-5-(3-fluorophenyl)-1,3,4-oxadiazole; 3-fluro-				
Toluene	6	375 (BB)	N_2 (3 ns)		253

#M464 2-(1-Naphthyl)-5-(m-tolyl)-1,3,4-oxadiazole; 3-methyl-αNPD

Solvent	Conc.	Wavelength	Laser	Output	Ref.
Toluene	3.5	372 (BB)	N_2 (3 ns)		253

#M465 2,5-Bis(4-biphenylyl)-1,3,4-oxadiazole; BBD

Solvent	Conc.	Wavelength	Laser	Output	Ref.
Xylene	Satur.	374–397.8 (grating)	N_2 (100 kW)		194
Toluene	3.5	372–406.5 (grating)	N_2 (270 kW)	78 kW	220
Dioxane	2	372–405 (grating)	N_2 (530 kW, 3.5 ns)	E = 19.3%	139
Dioxane	2	376.7 (BB)	Fl (81.5 J, 80 ns, RT)	15.6 mJ, 220 kW	179
Dioxane	1	375.6 (BB)	XeCl (60 mJ, 35 ns)	E = 13.7%	95

#M466 2-(1-Biphenyl)-5-(1-naphthyl)-1,3,4-oxadiazole; αNBD

Solvent	Conc.	Wavelength	Laser	Output	Ref.
Toluene	5	383–386.5 (BB)	N_2		254

#M467 2-(1-Biphenyl)-5-(2-naphthyl)-1,3,4-oxadiazole; βNBD

Solvent	Conc.	Wavelength	Laser	Output	Ref.
Toluene	5	372.2–375.8 (BB)	N_2		254

(continued)

Table 28 *(continued)*

Solvent	Concentration (mM)	Lasing wavelength (tuning) (nm)	Excitation	Output	Ref.
#M468 2,5-Bis(1-naphthyl)-1,3,4-oxadiazole; αNND					
Toluene	3.1	391 (BB)	Nd-TH (8 MW)	E = 6.5%	177
Benzene	3.1	391 (BB)	Nd-TH (7 MW)	E = 4.5%	
Toluene	4	385-417 (grating)	N$_2$ (270 kW)	73 kW	220
#M469 2-(1-Naphthyl)-5-styryl-1,3,4-oxadiazole					
Toluene	0.01-1	399 (BB)	Nd-TH (0.04 J, 40 ns)		168
PMMA		416 (BB)			
#M470 2-Biphenylyl-5-styryl-1,3,4-oxadiazole					
Toluene	3.1	390.5 (BB)	Nd-TH (8 MW)	E = 2.5%	177
Benzene	3.1	391.5 (BB)	Nd-TH (7.5 MW)	E = 3.5%	

#M471 *p*-Bis(5-phenyl-1,3,4-oxadiazole-2-yl)benzene; PDPDP

| Dioxane | 2 | 416–452 (grating) | N_2 (530 kW, 3.5 ns) | E = 17.7% | 139 |

---

[a] Chemical structures of oxadiazole derivatives. The symbols (a)–(i) are shown in Table 29.

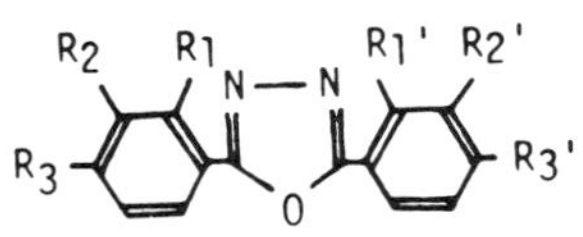

#M439- #M453

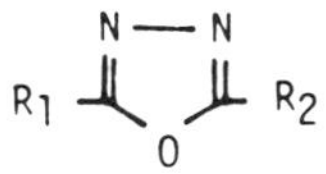

#M454, #M458

#M455- #M457,

#M459- #M470

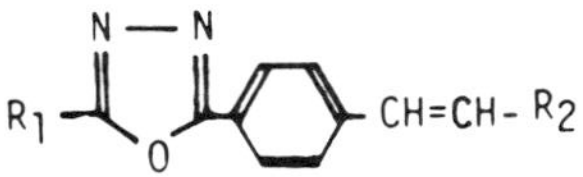

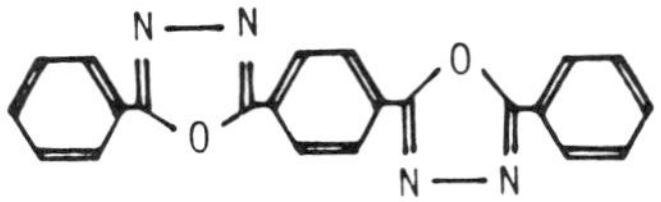

#M471

Table 28 (continued)

Dye no.	R1	R2	R3	R1	R2	R3
#M439	H	H	H	H	H	H
#M440	F	H	H	H	H	H
#M441	H	F	H	H	H	H
#M442	H	H	F	H	H	H
#M443	H	H	Br	H	H	H
#M444	Cl	H	Cl	H	H	H
#M445	H	Cl	Cl	H	H	H
#M446	H	H	OCH$_3$	H	H	H
#M447	H	H	NMe$_2$	H	H	H
#M448	F	H	H	F	H	H
#M449	H	F	H	H	F	H
#M450	H	H	Cl	H	H	Cl
#M451	H	H	OCH$_3$	H	H	OCH$_3$
#M452	H	H	NEt$_2$	H	H	NEt$_2$
#M453	H	H	NMe$_2$	H	H	Cl

Dye no.	R1	R2
#M455	Ph	(d)
#M456	(a); X = Bu	(d)
#M457	(a); X = iso-Pr	(d)
#M458	(d)	Ph
#M459	Ph	(c)
#M460	(a); X = OCH$_3$	(c)
#M461	(a); X = Br	(c)
#M462	(h)	(c)
#M463	(i); X = F	(c)
#M464	(i); X = Me	(c)
#M465	(d)	(d)
#M466	(d)	(c)
#M467	(d)	(e)
#M468	(c)	(c)
#M469	(c)	(g)

Table 29. Laser Characteristics of Furan and Benzofuran Derivatives[a,b]

Solvent	Concentration (mM)	Lasing wavelength (tuning) (nm)	Excitation	Output	Ref.
		#M472 2,5-Diphenylfuran; PPF			
Benzene or ethanol	1-10	369-379.5 (BB, concentration + solvent)	N_2 (20-40 kW, 10 Hz)		232
Ethanol		365-371 (grating)	N_2 (100 kW, 10 ns, 100 Hz)		185
DMF	0.4	371 (BB)	Fl (20 J, 50 ns, RT)	Thr = 11 J	137
Dioxane		371 (BB)		Thr = 10 J	
Xylene	5	370.2-377.6 (grating)	N_2 (100 kW)		194
Toulene	1.5	366.5-380 (grating)	N_2 (270 kW)	65 kW	220

(continued)

Table 29 *(continued)*

Solvent	Concentration (mM)	Lasing wavelength (tuning) (nm)	Excitation	Output	Ref.
		#M473 1,3-Diphenylisobenzofuran			
Ethanol (de-oxgenated)	75 mg/l	484–518 (grating)	Fl (100 J, 800 ns, RT)		74
Ethanol + COT	0.2		Fl (120 J, 1.5 µs, RT)	(5.9 µs)	
Ethanol	0.3	500 (BB)	Fl (28 J, 200 ns, RT, 20 Hz)	1 mJ (20 Hz)	255
Ethanol		485–515 (prism, ring cavity, single axial mode)	Fl (60 J)	8 kW	101

[a] Structures:

#M472

#M473

[b]Lately laser action in five new furan derivatives (2-amino-4-cyano-3,5-diarylfuran) was reported in the blue-violet region (see Ref. 314).

Table 30. Laser Characteristics of Pyrazoline Derivatives[a]

Solvent	Concentration (mM)	Lasing wavelength (tuning) (nm)	Excitation	Ref.
#M474 1-m-Chlorophenyl-3-phenyl-2-pyrazoline				
Methanol	1	516 (BB)	N_2 (1 MW, 2.5 ns)	155
#M475 3-p-Chlorophenyl-5-phenyl-1-p-sulfophenyl-2-pyrazoline				
Methanol (base)	1	544 (BB)	N_2 (1 MW, 2.5 ns)	155
#M476 1,5-Diphenyl-3-styryl-2-pyrazoline				
PMMA	0.01-1	450 (BB)	Nd-TH (0.04 J, 40 ns)	168
#M477 3-p-Chlorostyryl-1,5-diphenyl-2-pyrazoline				
PMMA	0.01-1	457 (BB)	Nd-TH (0.04 J, 40 ns)	168

[a]Structures:

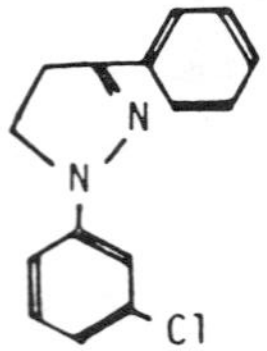

#M474

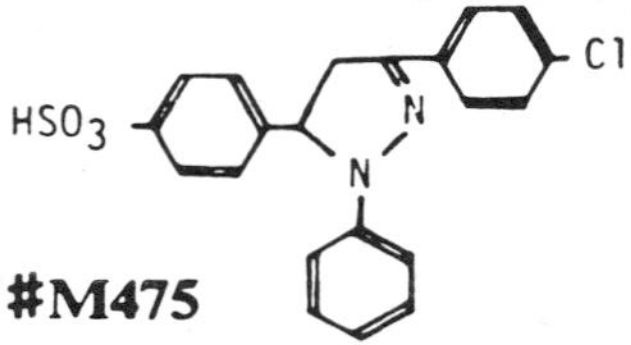

#M475

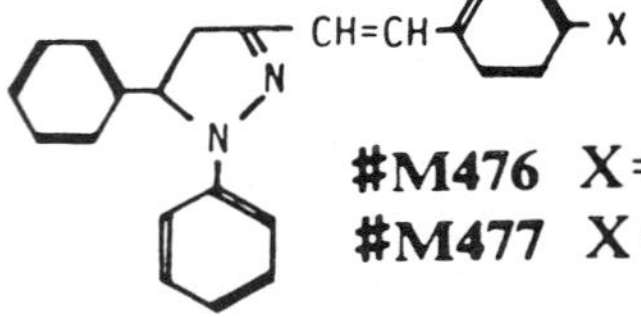

#M476 X=H; #M477 X=Cl

Table 31. Laser Characteristics of Phthalimide and Naphthalimide Derivatives[a]

Solvent	Concentration (mM)	Lasing wavelength (tuning) (nm)	Excitation	Output	Ref.
		#M478 3-Aminophthalimide			
Isoamyl alcohol		500 (BB)	Ruby-SH		2
		#M479 3-Amino-N-methylphthalimide			
Ethanol	10^{18} cm^{-3}	519 (BB)	Ruby-SH		258
Ethanol + DBT	$2 + 1$	504 (BB)	Fl (380 J, 30μs)	3 mJ	81
		#M480 4-Amino-N-methylphthalimide			
Dioxane + water or ethanol (1-50%)		476-538 (BB, solvent)	Ruby-SH		259

(continued)

Table 31 *(continued)*

Solvent	Concentration (mM)	Lasing wavelength (tuning) (nm)	Excitation	Output	Ref.
#M481 3,6-Diamino-*N*-methylphthalimide					
Vapor		~550 (BB)	Laser pump (pulse)		260
Propanol (-100 ~ 50°C)		(BB)	Fl		261
#M482 3-Acetylamino-6-amino-*N*-methylphthalimide					
Ethanol + DPB	1 + 5	546 (BB)	Fl (380 J, 30 μs)	30 mJ	81
#M483 3-Dimethylamino-6-methylamino-*N*-methylphthalimide					
Glycerin		610 (BB)	Nd-SH		122
Ethanol		595 (BB)	Nd-SH		
#M484 3,6-Tetramethyldiamino-*N*-methylphthalimide					
Ethanol		584 (BB)	Nd-SH		122
Cyclohexane		578 (BB)			

#M485 4-Amino-1,8-naphthalimide

Solvent	Concentration	Tuning range	Pump (energy)	Output	Ref.
Methanol + coumarin 450 (+ COT, deoxygenated)	0.15 + 0.13	530–575 (BB)	Fl (73 J)	10 mJ, Thr = 43 J	100

#M486 4-Amino-3-sulfo-N-p-tolylnaphthalimide sodium salt; brilliant sulfoflavine

Solvent	Concentration	Tuning range	Pump (energy)	Output	Ref.
Ethanol (de-oxygenated)	120 mg/l	508–573 (grating)	Fl (200 J)		74
Ethanol	0.4	540 (BB)	Fl (18 J, 200 ns, RT, 20 Hz)	10 mWav.	255
Ethanol + DAMC (5 mM methanol) 1:25	Satur.	465–494 (prism + grating)	N_2 (130 kW)	16.5 kW	13
Ethanol		510–570 (prism) (ring cavity, single axial mode)	Fl (60 J)	1.5 kW	101

(continued)

Table 31 (continued)

Solvent	Concentration (mM)	Lasing wavelength (tuning) (nm)	Excitation	Output	Ref.
Ethanol + COT (de-oxygenated)	0.7	547 (BB)	Fl (1.7 kJ, 1.7 μs)	0.6 J	91
		520–620 (grating)	Fl (10 Hz)	0.8 Wav. (1.4 μs)	126

[a] Structures:

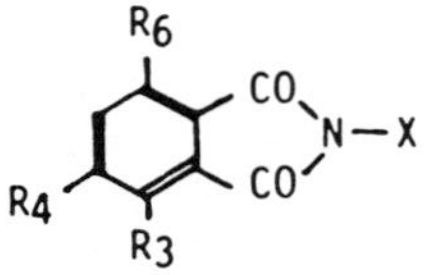

#M478- #M484

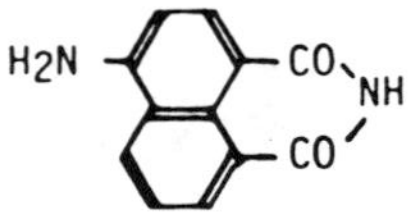

#M485

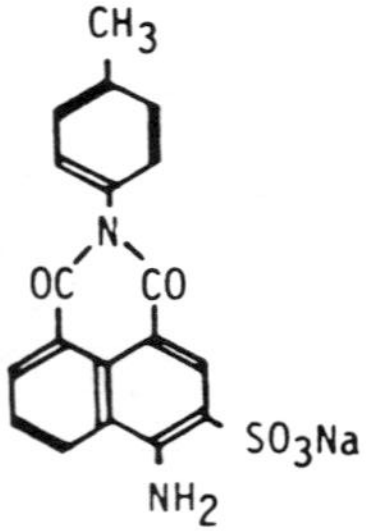

#M486

Dye no.	R_3	R_4	R_6	X
#M478	NH_2	H	H	H
#M479	NH_2	H	H	Me
#M480	H	NH_2	H	Me
#M481	NH_2	H	NH_2	Me
#M482	$NHCOCH_3$	H	NH_2	Me
#M483	NMe_2	H	$NHMe$	Me
#M484	NMe_2	H	NMe_2	Me

Table 32. Laser Characteristics of Pteridine Derivatives[a]

Solvent	Concentration (mM)	Lasing wavelength (tuning) (nm)	Excitation	Ref.
#M487 2-Amino-6,7-dimethyl-3,4-dihydropteridine-4-one				
Methanol (base)	1	460 (BB)	N_2 (1 MW, 2.5 ns)	155
#M488 7-Hydroxy-1,3,6-trimethyl-1,2,3,4-tetrahydropteridine-2,4-dione				
Methanol	1	375-380 (BB)	N_2 (1 MW, 2.5 ns)	155
#M489 Pteridine 1				
Water (base)	1	522 (BB)	N_2 (1 MW, 2.5 ns)	155
#M490 Pteridine 2				
Water (base)	Satur.	522 (BB)	N_2 (1 MW, 2.5 ns)	155

[a] Structures:

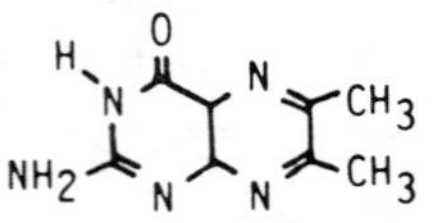

#M487

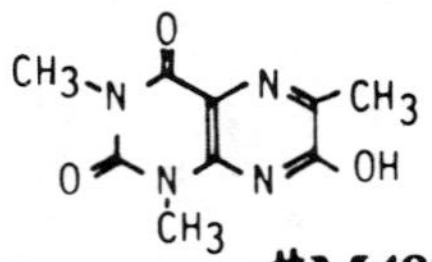

#M488

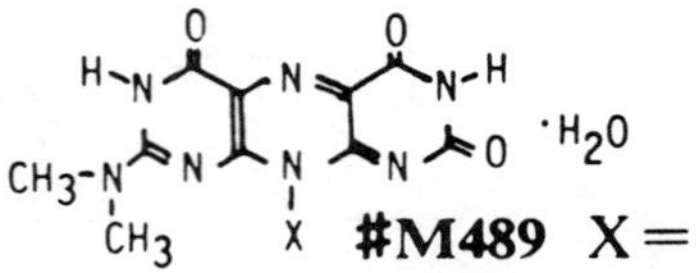

#M489 X=CH$_2$CH$_2$OH;
#M490 X=Me

Table 33. Laser Characteristics of Heterocyclic salts[a]

Solvent	Concentration (mM)	Lasing wavelength (tuning) (nm)	Excitation	Output	Ref.
		#M491 2,6-Diphenylpyrylium fluoborate			
Dichloro- methane	6	483 (BB)	N_2 (1 MW, 2.5 ns)		155
		#M492 2,4,6-Triphenylpyrylium fluoborate			
Methanol	1.7	485 (BB)	Ruby-SH (200 kW)		24
Dichloro- methane	1	468 (BB)	N_2 (1 MW, 2.5 ns)		155
		#M493 2-(p-Chlorophenyl)-4,6-diphenylpyrylium fluoborate			
Dichloro- methane	3	497 (BB)	N_2 (1 MW, 2.5 ns)		155
		#M494 4-(p-Chlorophenyl)-2,6-diphenylpyrylium fluoborate			
Dichloro- methane	1	492 (BB)	N_2 (1 MW, 2.5 ns)		155

(continued)

Table 33 (continued)

Solvent	Concentration (mM)	Lasing wavelength (tuning) (nm)	Excitation	Output	Ref.
#M495 2,4-Bis(p-chlorophenyl)-6-phenylpyrylium fluoborate					
Dichloro-methane	Satur.	501 (BB)	N_2 (1 MW, 2.5 ns)		155
#M496 2,6-Bis(p-chlorophenyl)-4-phenylpyrylium fluoborate					
Dichloro-methane	Satur.	505 (BB)	N_2 (1 MW, 2.5 ns)		155
#M497 2,4,6-Tris(p-chlorophenyl)pyrylium fluoborate					
Dichloro-methane	2	512 (BB)	N_2 (1 MW, 2.5 ns)		155
#M498 2,4,6-Tris(p-dimethylaminophenyl)pyrylium fluoborate					
Dichloro-methane	3	670 (BB)	N_2 (1 MW, 2.5 ns)		155

Solvent	Compound	λ (BB)		Pump	Ref.
Methanol	#M499 2,4,6-Tris(p-tolyl)pyrylium perchlorate	492 (BB)		Ruby-SH	52
Methanol	#M500 2,6-Bis(p-methoxyphenyl)-4-phenylpyrylium fluoborate	566–573		Ruby-SH, Fl	52
Dichloro-methane	#M501 2,6-Diphenyl-4-methylpyrylium fluoborate	475 (BB)	2	N_2 (1 MW, 2.5 ns)	155
Dichloro-methane	#M502 4-Carboxy-2,6-diphenylpyrylium fluoborate	522 (BB)	3	N_2 (1 MW, 2.5 ns)	155
Dichloro-methane	#M503 4-Carbethoxy-2,6-diphenylpyrylium fluoborate	526 (BB)	3	N_2 (1 MW, 2.5 ns)	155
Dichloro-methane	#M504 4-Butyryl-2,6-diphenylpyrylium fluoborate	527 (BB)	3	N_2 (1 MW, 2.5 ns)	155

(continued)

Table 33 *(continued)*

Solvent	Concentration (mM)	Lasing wavelength (tuning) (nm)	Excitation	Output	Ref.
#M505 2,4-Diphenyl-6-methylpyrylium fluoborate					
Dichloro-methane	1	448 (BB)	N$_2$ (1 MW, 2.5 ns)		155
#M506 2-Carboxy-4,6-diphenylpyrylium fluoborate					
Dichloro-methane	3	488 (BB)	N$_2$ (1 MW, 2.5 ns)		155
#M507 2,4-Diphenyl-6-styrylpyrylium fluoborate					
Dichloro-methane	3	560 (BB)	N$_2$ (1 MW, 2.5 ns)		155
#M508 4-Carboxy-2,6-bis(*p*-methoxybenzyl)pyrylium fluoborate					
Dichloro-methane	1	623 (BB)	N$_2$ (1 MW, 2.5 ns)		155

#M509 4-Carbethoxy-2,6-Bis(*p*-methoxybenzyl)pyrylium fluoborate	Dichloromethane	3 (BB)	631	N_2 (1 MW, 2.5 ns)	155
#M510 2,4,6-Tris(*p*-methoxybenzyl)pyrylium fluoborate	Dichloromethane	3 (BB)	545	N_2 (1 MW, 2.5 ns)	155
#M511 2,6-Bis(2-thienyl)-4-phenylpyrylium fluoborate	Dichloromethane	3 (BB)	550	N_2 (1 MW, 2.5 ns)	155
#M512 Pyryliumsalt 1	Dichloromethane	Satur. (BB)	524	N_2 (1 MW, 2.5 ns)	155
#M513 Pyryliumsalt 2	Dichloromethane	3 (BB)	497	N_2 (1 MW, 2.5 ns)	155
#M514 Pyryliumsalt 3	Dichloromethane	3 (BB)	515	N_2 (1 MW, 2.5 ns)	155

(*continued*)

Table 33 *(continued)*

Solvent	Concentration (mM)	Lasing wavelength (tuning) (nm)	Excitation	Output	Ref.
#M515 Pyryliumsalt 4					
Dichloro-methane	3	532 (BB)	N_2 (1 MW, 2.5 ns)		155
#M516 Pyryliumsalt 5					
Dichloro-methane	3	534	N_2 (1 MW, 2.5 ns)		155
#M517 Pyryliumsalt 6					
Dichloro-methane	3	478 (BB)	N_2 (1 MW, 2.5 ns)		155
#M518 Pyryliumsalt 7					
Dichloro-methane	3	532 (BB)	N_2 (1 MW, 2.5 ns)		155

#M519 Pyryliumsalt 8

Solvent				
Dichloromethane	3	627 (BB)	N_2 (1 MW, 2.5 ns)	155

#M520 Pyryliumsalt 9

Dichloromethane	3	508 (BB)	N_2 (1 MW, 2.5 ns)	155

#M521 Pyryliumsalt 10; DMX

Acetonitryl	$5 \times 10^{15} - 10^{18}$ cm^{-3}	600–622 (BB, concentration)	Fl	Thr = 50 J	262

#M522 Pyryliumsalt 11; DMC

Acetonitryl	$10^{16} - 2 \times 10^{17}$ cm^{-3}	606–616 (BB, concentration)	Fl	Thr = 300 J	262

#M523 2,4,6-Triphenyl-1,3-oxazin-1-ium fluoborate

Dichloromethane	2	442 (BB)	N_2 (1 MW, 2.5 ns)	155

#M524 2,6-Diphenylthiapyrylium perchlorate

Dichloromethane	3	513 (BB)	N_2 (1 MW, 2.5 ns)	155

(continued)

Table 33 (*continued*)

Solvent	Concentration (mM)	Lasing wavelength (tuning) (nm)	Excitation	Output	Ref.
#M525 2,4-Diphenyl-6-(*p*-methoxybenzyl) thiapyrylium perchlorate					
Dichloro-methane	3	618 (BB)	N$_2$ (1 MW, 2.5 ns)		155
#M526 2,6-Bis(*p*-methoxybenzyl)-4-phenylthiapyrylium fluoborate					
Dichloro-methane	2	612 (BB)	N$_2$ (1 MW, 2.5 ns)		155
#M527 2,4,6-Tris(*p*-methoxybenzyl) thiapyrylium perchlorate					
Dichloro-methane	3	601 (BB)	N$_2$ (1 MW, 2.5 ns)		155
#M528 1,1-Dimethoxy-2,4,6-tris(*p*-tolyl) phosphorin					
Benzene	3	529 (BB)	N$_2$ (1 MW, 2.5 ns)		155
#M529 1,1-Dimethoxy-2,6-diphenyl-4-*p*-methoxybenzyl phosphorin					
Benzene	3	536 (BB)	N$_2$ (1 MW, 2.5 ns)		155

#M530 Bis(1,1-Dimethoxy-2,6-diphenylphosphorin-4-yl) methane

Benzene	3	522 (BB)	N$_2$ (1 MW, 2.5 ns)		155

#M531 Spiro-2-[3-methyl-2,1,3-oxazaphospholidine]-1-[2,4,6-triphenylphosphorin]

Benzene	3	502 (BB)	N$_2$ (1 MW, 2.5 ns)		155

#M532 Boratriazinium salt

Dichloro-methane	Satur.	420 (BB)	N$_2$ (1 MW, 2.5 ns)		155

#M533 Boradiazinium salt

DMF	Satur.	565 (BB)	N$_2$ (1 MW, 2.5 ns)		155

#M534 2,6-Diaminopyridine hydroperchlorate

Ethanol (acid)		391-403 (BB)	Fl (200 ns, RT)	Thr = 28 J	184

#M535 2,6-Bis(methylamino)pyridine hydroperchlorate

Ethanol (acid)		409-423 (BB)	Fl (200 ns, RT)	Thr = 32 J	184

(continued)

Table 33 (*continued*)

Solvent	Concentration (mM)	Lasing wavelength (tuning) (nm)	Excitation	Output	Ref.
#M536 2,6-Bis(dimethylamino)pyridine hydroperchlorate					
Ethanol (acid)		434–440 (BB)	Fl (200 ns, RT)	Thr = 60 J	184

[a] Structures [symbols (1)–(7) are shown in Table 34].

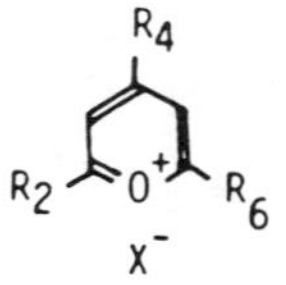

#M491- #511

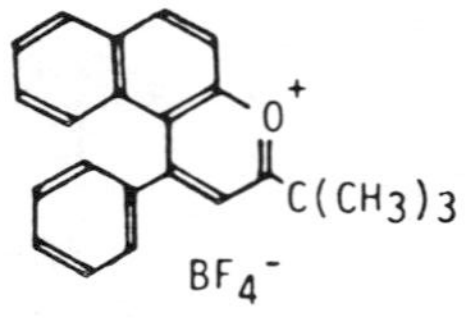

#M512

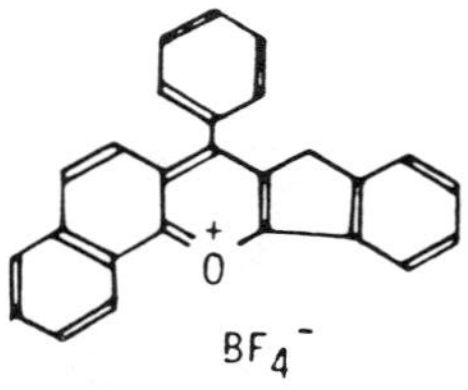

#M513

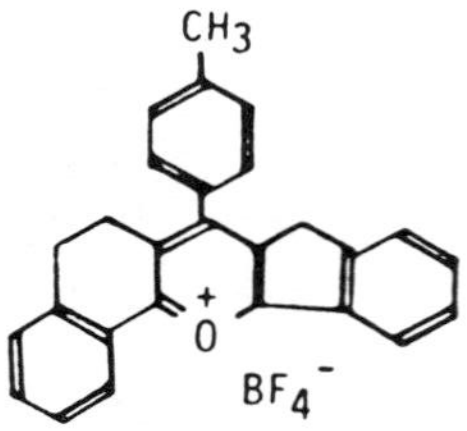

#M514

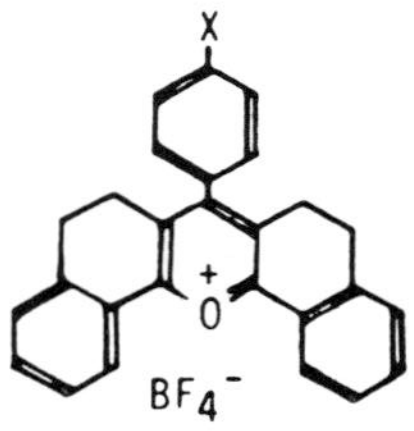

#M515 X=H; #M516 X=Me

#M517 X=Cl

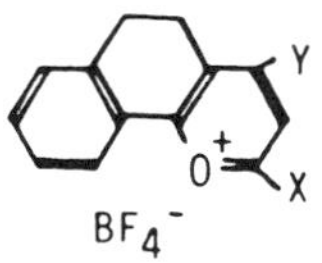

#M522 (estimated)

CHOC$_2$H$_5$

C1O$_4^-$

H$_5$C$_2$OHC

#M521 (estimated)

CHOC$_2$H$_5$

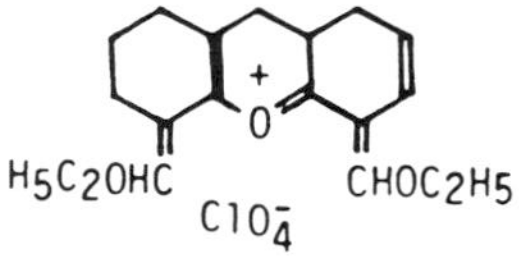

C1O$_4^-$

H$_5$C$_2$OHC

#M530

OCH$_3$
P—OCH$_3$

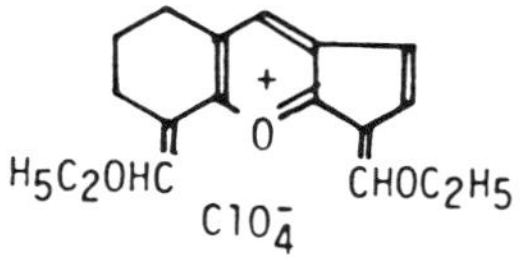

CH$_3$O—P
CH$_3$O

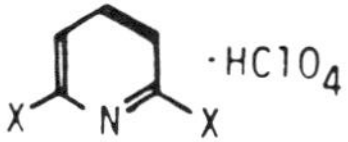

#M534 X=NH$_2$; #M535 X=NHMe
#M536 X=NMe$_2$

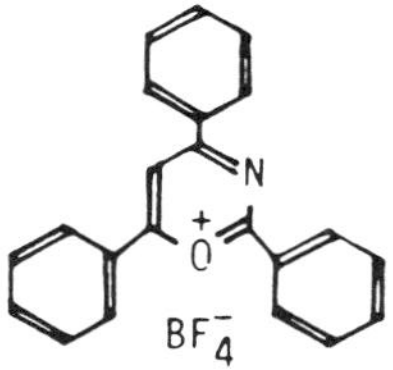

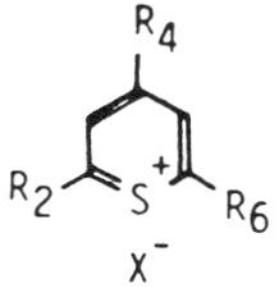

·HClO$_4$

#M528 ; #M529

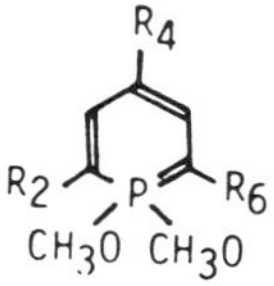

R$_4$

R$_2$ P   R$_6$
CH$_3$O CH$_3$O

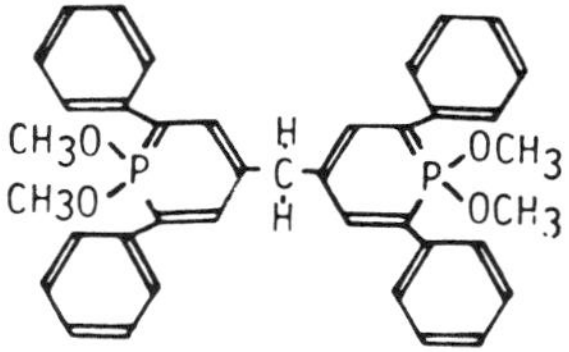

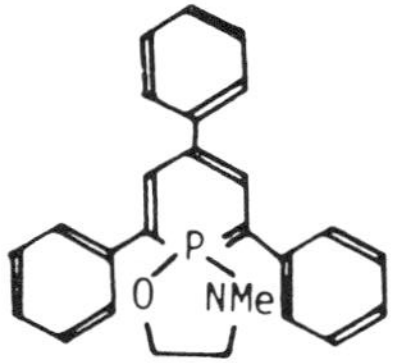

#M520

BF$_4^-$

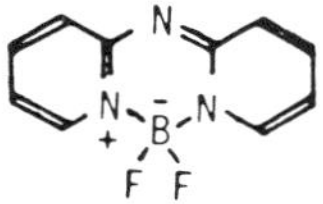

#M524- #M527

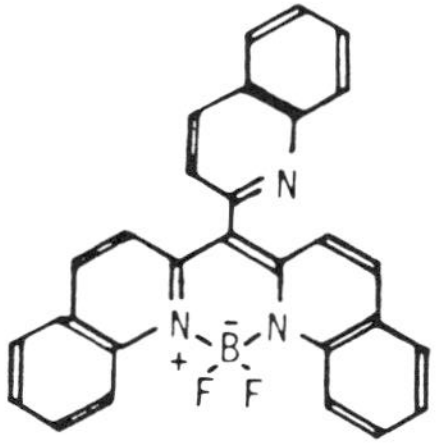

R$_4$

R$_2$ S$^+$ R$_6$
X$^-$

#M533

#M518 X=Bu, Y=p-Tolyl
#M519 X=Ph, Y=Ph

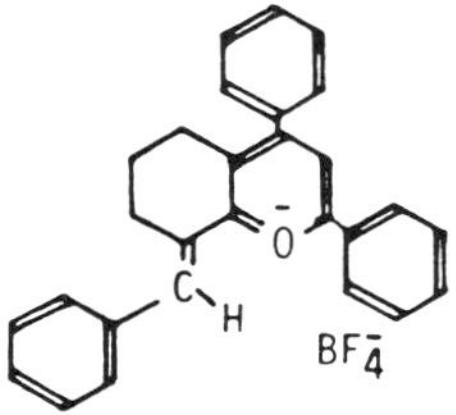

BF$_4^-$

#M523

BF$_4^-$

#M532

#M531

NMe

P
O

(continued)

Table 33 (*continued*)

Dye no.	R_2	R_4	R_6	X
#M491	Ph	H	Ph	BF_4
#M492	Ph	Ph	Ph	BF_4
#M493	Ph	Ph	(1)	BF_4
#M494	Ph	(1)	Ph	BF_4
#M495	(1)	(1)	Ph	BF_4
#M496	(1)	Ph	(1)	BF_4
#M497	(1)	(1)	(1)	BF_4
#M498	(2)	(2)	(2)	BF_4
#M499	(3)	(3)	(3)	ClO_4
#M500	(4)	Ph	(4)	BF_4
#M501	Ph	Me	Ph	BF_4
#M502	Ph	COOH	Ph	BF_4
#M503	Ph	$COOC_2H_5$	Ph	BF_4
#M504	Ph	COC_3H_7	Ph	BF_4
#M505	Ph	Ph	Me	BF_4
#M506	Ph	Ph	COOH	BF_4
#M507	Ph	Ph	(5)	ClO_4
#M508	(6)	COOH	(6)	BF_4
#M509	(6)	$COOC_2H_5$	(6)	BF_4
#M510	(6)	(6)	(6)	BF_4
#M511	(7)	Ph	(7)	BF_4
#M524	Ph	H	Ph	ClO_4
#M525	Ph	Ph	(6)	ClO_4
#M526	(6)	Ph	(6)	BF_4
#M527	(6)	(6)	(6)	ClO_4
#M528	(3)	(3)	(3)	—
#M529	Ph	(6)	Ph	—

Table 34. Abbreviations Used in Table 33

(1)   (2)   (3)   (4)

(5)   (6)   (7)

Table 35. Laser Characteristics of Other Heterocyclic Compounds[a]

Solvent	Concentration (mM)	Lasing wavelength (tuning) (nm)	Excitation	Ref.
#M537 Furanopyrone derivative				
Dichloromethane	Satur.	485 and 510 (BB)	N_2 (1 MW, 2.5 ns)	155
#M538 Morin; 2',3,4',5,7-pentahydroxyflavone				
Water + DMSO (2:8) + AlCl$_3$	6.72 + 6 g/l	523 (BB)	N_2 (2 mJ)	263
#M539 Xanthene dye N92				
Benzene	1	503 (BB)	N_2 (1 MW, 2.5 ns)	155
#M540 Xanthene dye N89				
Benzene	1	510 (BB)	N_2 (1 MW, 2.5 ns)	155
#M541 Thioxanthene dye N90				
Benzene	1	545 (BB)	N_2 (1 MW, 2.5 ns)	155
#M542 7-Ethoxy-3-phenylcoumarin				
Ethanol		478 (BB)	Nd-TH	264

#M543 3-Acetylumbelliferone

Ethanol	460 (BB)	Nd–TH	264

#M544 3-(4-Chloropyrazol-1-yl) umbelliferone

Ethanol	471 (BB)	Nd–TH	264

#M545 3-(1*H*-1,2,4-Triazol-1-yl) umbelliferone

Ethanol	472 (BB)	Nd–TH	264

#M546 3-(2-Benzothiazolyl)umbelliferone

Ethanol	517 (BB)	Nd–TH	264

---

[a] Structures (#M542–46 should be listed in Tables 23 and 24):

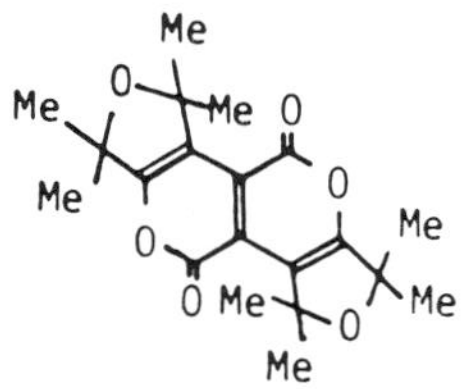

#M537

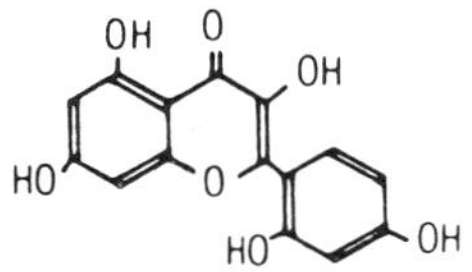

#M538

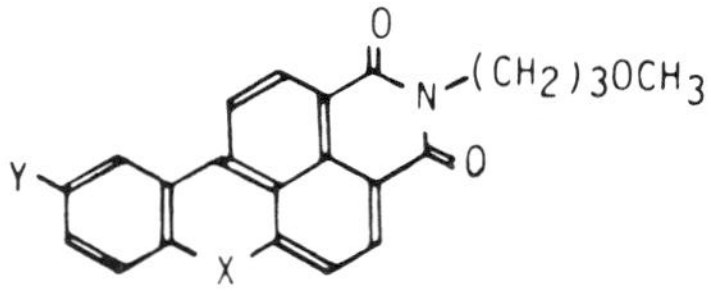

#M539 X=O, Y=H;
#M540 X=O, Y=OCH₃;
#M541 X=S, Y=H

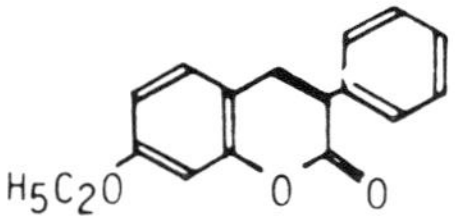

#M542

(continued)

Table 35 *(continued)*

#M543

#M544

#M545

#M546

References

1. M. Maeda and Y. Miyazoe: *Jpn. J. Appl. Phys.* **11**, 692 (1972).
2. B. I. Stepanov and A. N. Rubinov: *Sov. Phys. Usp.* **11**, 304 (1968).
3. Y. Miyazoe and M. Maeda: *Appl. Phys. Lett.* **12**, 206 (1968).
4. M. Maeda, K. Banno, and Y. Ogo: *Nippon Kanko-Shikiso Kenkyusho Hokoku* No. 46 (1974); Y. Miyazoe and M. Maeda: *Opto-Electronics (London)* **2**, 227 (1970).
5. M. L. Spaeth and D. P. Bortfeld: *Appl. Phys. Lett.* **9**, 179 (1966).
6. B. I. Stepanov, A. N. Rubinov, and V. A. Mostovnikov: *JETP Lett. (Engl. Transl.)* **5**, 117 (1967).
7. A. M. Bonch-Bruevich, N. N. Zatsepina, T. K. Razumova, G. M. Rubanova, I. F. Tupitsin, and V. N. Shuvalova: *Opt. Spektrosk.* **28**, 51 (1970).
8. O. V. Przhonskaya and E. A. Tikhonov: *Opt. Specktrosk.* **44**, 280 (1978).
9. F. P. Schäfer, W. Schmidt, and J. Volze: *Appl. Phys. Lett.* **9**, 306 (1966).
10. G. Carboni, A. DiBene, G. Gorini, E. Polacco, and G. Torelli: *Lett. Nuovo Ciment Soc. Ital. Fis.* **1**, 979 (1971).
11. A. Hirth and K. Vollrath: *Opt. Commun.* **7**, 339 (1973).
12. P. K. Runge: *Opt. Commun.* **5**, 311 (1972).
13. E. D. Stokes, F. B. Dunning, R. F. Stebbings, G. K. Walters, and R. D. Rundel: *Opt. Commun.* **5**, 267 (1972).
14. F. B. Dunning and E. D. Stokes: *Opt. Commun.* **6**, 160 (1972).
15. C. E. Hackett and C. F. Dewey, Jr.: *IEEE J. Quantum. Electron.* **QE–9**, 1119 (1973).
16. O. Hildebrand: *Opt. Commun.* **10**, 310 (1974).
17. C. Lin: *J. Appl. Phys.* **46**, 4076 (1975).
18. K. M. Romanek, O. Hildebrand, and E. Göbel: *Opt. Commun.* **21**, 16 (1977).
19. R. Mahon, T. J. McIlrath, and D. W. Koopman: *Appl. Opt.* **18**, 891 1979).
20. P. E. Oettinger and C. F. Dewey, Jr.: *IEEE J. Quantum Electron.* **QE–12**, 95 (1976).

21. G. Yamaguchi, S. Murakawa, and C. Yamanaka: *Technol. Rep. Osaka Univ.* **18**, 425 (1968).
22. L. D. Derkacheva, A. I. Krymova, A. F. Vompe, and I. I. Levkoev: *Opt. Spektrosk. (Engl. Transl.)*, **25**, 404 (1968).
23. C. Lin: *IEEE J. Quantum Electron.* **QE–11**, 61 (1975).
24. F. P. Schäfer, W. Schmidt, and K. Marth: *Phys. Lett.* **24A**, 280 (1967).
25. C. Rulliere: *Chem. Phys. Lett.* **43**, 303 (1976).
26. "Catalogue of Lambda Physik" D3400, Göttingen, Postfach 204, Germany.
27. J. S. Bakos and Zs. Sörlei: *Opt. Commun.* **22**, 258 (1977).
28. D. J. Bradley, A. J. F. Durrant, G. M. Gale, M. Moore, and P. D. Smith: *IEEE J. Quantum Electron.* **QE–4**, 707 (1968).
29. P. P. Sorokin, W. H. Culver, E. C. Hammond, and J. R. Lankard: *IBM J. Res. Dev.* **10**, 401 (1966).
30. P. P. Sorokin, J. R. Lankard, E. C. Hammond, and V. L. Moruzzi: *IBM J. Res. Dev.* **11**, 130 (1967).
31. C. D. Decker and F. K. Tittel: *Opt. Commun.* **7**, 155 (1973).
32. J. P. Webb, F. G. Webster, and B. E. Plourde: *IEEE J. Quantum Electron.* **QE–11**, 114 (1975).
33. K. Kato: *IEEE J. Quantum Electron.* **QE–12**, 442 (1976).
34. A Passner and T. Venkatesan: *Rev. Sci. Instrum.* **49**, 1413 (1978).
35. J. M. Yarborough: *Appl. Phys. Lett.* **24**, 629 (1974).
36. K. Kato: *Opt. Commun.* **19**, 18 (1976).
37. C. Loth, Y. H. Meyer, and F. Bos: *Opt. Commun.* **16**, 310 (1976).
38. C. Loth and P. Flamant: *Opt. Commun.* **21**, 13 (1977).
39. J. Kuhl, R. Lambrich, and D. V. der Linde: *Appl. Phys. Lett.* **31**, 657 (1977).
40. J. Cahen, M. Clerc, and P. Rigny: *Opt. Commun.* **21**, 387 (1977).
41. "Catalogue of Spectra-Physics" (1250 W. Middlefield Road, Mountain View, California 94042).
42. C. D. Decker: *Appl. Phys. Lett.* **27**, 607 (1975).
43. A. Donzel and C. Weisbuch: *Opt. Commun.* **17**, 153 (1976).
44. H. Lotem: *Opt. Commun.* **9**, 346 (1973).
45. L. O. Hocker: *IEEE J. Quantum Electron.* **QE–13**, 548 (1977).
46. M. Leduc: *Opt. Commun.* **31**, 66 (1979).
47. S. Chandra, N. Takeuchi, and S. R. Hartmann: *Appl. Phys. Lett.* **21**, 144 (1972).
48. G. Wang: *Opt. Commun.* **10**, 149 (1974).
49. M. Leduc and C. Weisbuch: *Opt. Commun.* **26**, 78 (1978).
50. "Catalogue of General Electric, Space Sciences Lab."
51. L. D. Derkacheva, A. I. Krymova, V. I. Malyshev, and A. S. Markin: *JETP Lett. (Engl. Transl.)* **7**, 362 (1968).
52. V. F. P. Schäfer: *Angew. Chem.* **82**, 25 (1970).

53. K. Kato: *IEEE J. Quantum Electron* **QE–14**, 7 (1978).
54. J. L. Oudar, Ph. J. Kupecek, and D. S. Chemla: *Opt. Commun.* **29**, 119 (1979).
55. K. Kato: *Appl. Phys. Lett.* **33**, 509 (1978).
56. A. Ferrario: *Opt. Commun.* **30**, 83 (1979).
57. A. Ferrario: *Opt. Commun.* **30**, 85 (1979).
58. P. Varga, P. G. Kryukov, V. F. Kuprishov, and Yu. V. Senatskii: *JETP Lett.* (*Engl. Transl.*) **8**, 307 (1968).
59. H. Bücher and W. Chow: *Appl. Phys.* **13**, 267 (1977).
60. K. H. Drexhage and F. P. Schäfer: "Dye Lasers." Springer-Verlag, Berlin, 1973.
61. H. Kuhn: *J. Chem. Phys.* **17**, 1198 (1949).
62. G. E. Busch, K. S. Greve, G. L. Olson, R. P. Jones, and P. M. Rentzepis: *Chem. Phys. Lett.* **33**, 412, 415 (1975).
63. J. P. Fouassier, D. J. Lougnot, and J. Faure: *Opt. Commun.* **18**, 263 (1976).
64. V. A. Zaporozhchenko, A. N. Rubinov, and T. Sh. Efendiev: *Sov. Tech. Phys. Lett.* (*Engl. Transl.*) **3**, 46 (1977).
65. G. G. Dyadyusha, I. P. Il'chishin, Yu. L. Slominskii, E. A. Tikhonov, A. I. Tolmachev, and M. T. Shpak: *Sov. J. Quantum Electron.* (*Engl. Transl.*) **6**, 349 (1976).
66. R. S. Hargrove and T. Kan: *Conf. Laser Eng. Appl.* **7.1** (1977).
67. P. R. Hammond: *Opt. Commun.* **29**, 331 (1979).
68. R. Kugel, A. Svirmickas, J. J. Katz, and J. C. Hindman: *Opt. Commun.* **23**, 189 (1977).
69. P. P. Sorokin and J. R. Lankard: *IBM J. Res. Dev.* **10**, 162 (1966).
70. P. P. Sorokin and J. R. Lankard: *IBM J. Res. Dev.* **11**, 148 (1967).
71. L. R. Lidholt and W. W. Wladimiroff: *Opto-electronics* (*London*) **2**, 21 (1970).
72. Y. Imano, M. Takemura, T. Kobayashi, F. Inaba: *Rep. Quantum Electron. Meet. IECE Jpn.* **QE70–35** (1970).
73. K. Kato, A. J. Alcock, M. C. Richardson, T. Fujioka: *Oyōbutsuri* **42**, 574 (1973).
74. J. B. Marling, D. W. Gregg, and S. J. Thomas: *IEEE J. Quantum Electron.* **QE–6**, 570 (1970); J. B. Marling, D. W. Gregg, and L. Wood: *Appl. Phys. Lett.* **17**, 527 (1970).
75. W. Schmidt and F. P. Schäfer: *Z. Naturfor.* **22a**, 1563 (1967).
76. V. D. Kotsubanov, Yu. V. Naboikin, L. A. Ogurtsova, A. P. Podgornyi, and F. S. Pokrovskaya: *Opt. Spektrosk.* (*Engl. Transl.*) **25**, 159, 406 (1968).
77. V. D. Kotsubanov, Yu. V. Naboikin, L. A. Ogurtsova, A. P. Podgornyi, and F. S. Pokrovskaya: *Sov. Phys. Tech. Phys.* (*Engl. Trans.*) **13**, 923 (1969).
78. D. W. Gregg and S. J. Thomas: *IEEE J. Quantum Electron.* **QE–5**, 302 (1969).

79. B. C. Fawcett: *IEEE J. Quantum Electron.* **QE–6,** 473 (1970).
80. Y. Miyazoe and M. Maeda: *Technol. Rep. Kyushu Univ.* **41,** 773 (1968).
81. M. B. Levin, A. S. Cherkasov, and V. I. Shirokov: *Opt. Spektrosk. (Engl. Transl.)* **41,** 82 (1976).
82. S. A. Tuccio and F. C. Strome, Jr.: *Appl. Opt.* **11,** 64 (1972).
83. K. H. Drexhage *et al.: Laser Focus* **9,** 35 (1973).
84. S. M. Jarrett and J. F. Young: *Opt. Lett.* **4,** 176 (1979).
85. S. Sriram, H. E. Jackson, and J. T. Boyd: *Appl. Phys. Lett.* **36,** 721 (1980).
86. Catalogue of Coherent, Inc. (3210 Porter Drive, Palo Alto, California 94304).
87 "Catalogue of Phase-R Company" (Box G-2, Old Rt. 11, New Durham, New Hampshire 03855).
88. B. B. McFarland: *Appl. Phys. Lett.* **10,** 208 (1967).
89. E. G. Arthurs, D. J. Bradley, and A. G. Roddie: *Appl. Phys. Lett.* **20,** 125 (1972).
90. C. Loth and Y. H. Meyer: *Appl. Opt.* **12,** 123 (1973).
91. M. Maeda, T. Okada, K. Fujiwara, and Y. Miyazoe: *Proc. Annu. Meet. IEE Jpn. Kyushu,* p. 522 (1975).
92. W. Hartig: *Opt. Commun.* **27,** 447 (1978).
93. D. Huppert and P. M. Rentzepis: *J. Appl. Phys.* **49,** 543 (1978).
94. D. M. Guthals and J. W. Nibler: *Opt. Commun.* **29,** 322 (1979).
95. O. Uchino, T. Mizunami, M. Maeda, and Y. Miyazoe: *Appl. Phys.* **19,** 35 (1979).
96. E. R. Carney, D. W. Fahey, and L. D. Schearer: *IEEE J. Quantum Electron.* **QE–16,** 9 (1980).
97. "Catalogue of Molectron Corporation" (177 N. Wolfe Road, Sunnyvale, California 94086).
98. "Catalogue of Quanta-Ray" (2134 Old Middlefield Way, Mountain View, California 94043).
99. D. W. Gregg, M. R. Querry, J. B. Marling, S. J. Thomas, C. V. Dobler, N. J. Davies, and J. F. Belew: *IEEE J. Quantum Electron.* **QE–6,** 270 (1970).
100. J. B. Marling, J. G. Hawley, E. M. Liston, and W. B. Grant: *Appl. Opt.* **13,** 2317 (1974).
101. G. Marowsky: *IEEE J. Quantum Electron.* **QE–9,** 245 (1973).
102. P. P. Sorokin, J. R. Lankard, V. L. Moruzzi, and E. C. Hammond: *J. Chem. Phys.* **48,** 4726 (1968).
103. O. G. Peterson and B. B. Snavely: *Appl. Phys. Lett.* **12,** 238 (1968).
104. J. R. Lankard and R. J. Gutfeld: *IEEE J. Quantum Electron.* **QE–5,** 625 (1969).
105. R. Pappalardo, H. Samelson, and A. Lempicki: *IEEE J. Quantum Electron.* **QE–6,** 716 (1970).

106. O. G. Peterson, S. A. Tuccio, and B. B. Snavely: *Appl. Phys. Lett.* **17**, 245 (1970).
107. A. Dienes, E. P. Ippen, and C. V. Shank: *IEEE J. Quantum Electron.* **QE–8**, 388 (1972).
108. T. W. Hänsch, A. L. Schawlow, and P. Toschek: *IEEE J. Quantum Electron.* **QE–9**, 553 (1973).
109. C. M. Ferrar: *Appl. Phys. Lett.* **23**, 548 (1973).
110. P. Anliker, M. Gassmann, and H. Weber: *Opt. Commun.* **5**, 137 (1972).
111. F. N. Baltakov, B. A. Barikhin, and L. V. Sukhanov: *JETP Lett.* (*Engl. Transl.*) **19**, 174 (1974).
112. W. W. Morey and W. H. Glenn: *IEEE J. Quantum Electron.* **QE–12**, 311 (1976).
113. J. Jethwa, F. P. Schäfer, and J. Jasny: *IEEE J. Quantum Electron.* **QE–14**, 119 (1978).
114. C. H. Weysenfeld: *Appl. Opt.* **13**, 2816 (1974).
115. W. T. Silfvast and O. R. Wood: *Appl. Phys. Lett.* **26**, 447 (1975).
116. M. D. Levenson and G. L. Eesley: *IEEE J. Quantum Electron.* **QE–12**, 259 (1976).
117. P. Anliker, H. R. Lüthi, W. Seelig, J. Steinger, H. P. Weber, S. Leutwyler, E. Schumacher, and L. Wöste: *IEEE J. Quantum Electron.* **QE–13**, 547 (1977).
118. S. Kuroda and K. Kubota: *Appl. Phys. Lett.* **29**, 737 (1976).
119. J. R. Onstott: *Appl. Phys. Lett.* **31**, 818 (1977).
120. V. I. Tomin, A. J. Alcock, W. J. Sarjeant, and K. E. Leopold: *Opt. Commun.* **26**, 396 (1978).
121. C. V. Shank and E. P. Ippen: *Appl. Phys. Lett.* **24**, 373 (1974).
122. A. V. Aristov, E. N. Viktorova, D. A. Kozlovskii, and V. A. Kuzin: *Opt. Spektrosk.* (*Engl. Transl.*) **28**, 293 (1970).
123. L. A. Riseberg, A. Lempicki, H. Samelson, and R. M. Walters: *IEEE J. Quantum Electron.* **QE–10**, 132 (1974).
124. B. S. Neporent, V. B. Shilov, G. V. Lukomsky, and A. G. Spiro: *Chem. Phys. Lett.* **27**, 425 (1974).
125. J. Y. Allain: *Appl. Opt.* **18**, 287 (1979).
126. "Catalogue of Candela Corporation" (96 South Avenue, Natick, Massachusetts 01760).
127. B. W. Petley and K. Morris: *Opt. Quantum Electron.* **8**, 371 (1976).
128. K. Kato: *IEEE J. Quantum Electron.* **QE–13**, 544 (1977).
129. M. Yamashita, M. Kasamatsu, H. Kashiwagi, and K. Machida: *Opt. Commun.* **26**, 343 (1978).
130. J. A. Myer, C. L. Johnson, E. Kierstead, R. D. Sharma, and I. Itzkan: *Appl. Phys. Lett.* **16**, 3 (1970).
131. M. Hercher and H. A. Pike: *IEEE J. Quantum Electron.* **QE–7**, 473 (1971).

132. D. A. Jennings and A. J. Varga: *J. Appl. Phys.* **42**, 5171 (1971).
133. Y. Matsunaga, H. Ikeda, K. Matsumoto, and T. Fujioka: *J. Appl. Phys.* **48**, 842 (1977).
134. F. C. Strome, Jr. and S. A. Tuccio: *Opt. Commun.* **4**, 58 (1971).
135. P. R. Hammond: *J. Photochem.* **10**, 467 (1979).
136. P. R. Hammond and R. S. Hughes: *Nature (London) Phys. Sci.* **231**, 59 (1971).
137. H. W. Furumoto and H. L. Ceccon: *IEEE J. Quantum Electron.* **QE–6**, 262 (1970).
138. H. W. Furumoto and H. L. Ceccon: *J. Appl. Phys.* **40**, 4204 (1969).
139. M. Maeda and Y. Miyazoe: *Jpn. J. Appl. Phys.* **13**, 827 (1974).
140. K. Kato: *Opt. Commun.* **18**, 447 (1976).
141. C. A. Moore and L. S. Goldberg: *Opt. Commun.* **16**, 21 (1976).
142. J. Kuhl, H. Klingenberg, and D. Linde: *Appl. Phys.* **18**, 279 (1979).
143. K. H. Drexhage and G. A. Reynolds: *Int. Quantum Electron Conf.* **F.1** (1974).
144. F. A. Beisser and D. J. Eilenberger: *IEEE J. Quantum Electron.* **QE–11**, 372 (1975).
145. P. K. Runge: *Opt. Commun.* **4**, 195 (1971).
146. F. Castelli: *Appl. Phys. Lett.* **26**, 18 (1975).
147. D. Basting, D. Ouw, and F. P. Schäfer: *Opt. Commun.* **18**, 260 (1976).
148. V. I. Vashchuk, E. I. Zabello, and E. A. Tikhonov: *Sov. J. Quantum Electron.* (*Engl. Transl.*) **8**, 859 (1978).
149. U. Rebhan and J. Hildebrandt: *Opt. Commun.* **31**, 69 (1979).
150. G. W. Fehrenbach, K. J. Gruntz, and R. G. Ulbrich: *Appl. Phys. Lett.* **33**, 159 (1978).
151. J. C. Hindman, R. Kugel, A. Svirmickas, and J. J. Katz: *Proc. Natl. Acad. Sci. USA* **74**, 5 (1977).
152. "Catalogue of Exciton Chemical Company" (P.O. Box 3204, Overlock Station, Dayton, Ohio 45431).
153. R. J. Hall, J. A. Shirley, and A. C. Eckbreth: *Opt. Lett.* **4**, 87 (1979).
154. D. A. Fine and A. N. Fletcher: *Appl. Phys.* **13**, 287 (1977).
155. D. Basting, F. P. Schäfer, and B. Steyer: *Appl. Phys.* **3**, 81 (1974).
156. N. Karl: *Phys. Status Solidi A* **13**, 651 (1972).
157. N. Karl: *J. Lumin.* **12/13**, 851 (1976).
158. J. Ferguson and A. W. H. Mau: *Chem. Phys. Lett.* **14**, 245 (1972).
159. B. G. Huth and G. I. Farmer: *IEEE J. Quantum Electron.* **QE–4**, 427 (1968).
160. A. V. Aristov, V. A. Kuzin, and A. S. Cherkasov: *Opt. Spektrosk.* (*Engl. Transl.*) **35**, 192 (1973).
161. K. Tomioka and A. Matsui: *Jpn. J. Appl. Phys.* **19**, 1015 (1980).
162. J. R. Heldt and J. Heldt: *Acta Phys. Pol.* **A55**, 79 (1979).
163. B. Gronau, E. Lippert, and W. Rapp: *Ber. Bunsenges, Phys. Chem.*

76, 432 (1972).

164. C. Rulliere and M. M. Denariez-Roberge: *Opt. Commun.* **7,** 166 (1973).

165. K. H. Drexhage, G. R. Erikson, G. H. Hawks, and G. A. Reynolds: *Opt. Commun.* **15,** 399 (1975).

166. C. Rulliere, M. Laughrea, and M. M. Denariez-Roberge: *Opt. Commun.* **6,** 407 (1972).

167. I. B. Berlman, R. Rokni, and C. R. Goldschmidt: *Chem. Phys. Lett.* **22,** 458 (1973).

168. Yu. V. Naboikin, L. A. Ogurtsova, A. P. Podgornyi, F. S. Pokrovskaya, V. I. Grigoryeva, B. M. Krasovitskii, L. M. Kutsyna, and V. G. Tishchenko: *Opt. Spektrosk. (Engl. Transl.)* **28,** 528 (1970).

169. J. Kohlmannsperger: *Z. Naturforsch.* **24a,** 1547 (1969).

170. V. V. Danilov, A. S. Eremenko, Yu. T. Mazurenko, A. A. Rykov, Yu. L. Slominskii, and A. I. Stepanov: *Sov. J. Quantum Electron (Engl. Transl.)* **7,** 114 (1977).

171. A. V. Aristov, V. V. Danilov, L. K. Denisov, M. B. Levin, and V. N. Makarov: *Opt. Spektrosk. (Engl. Transl.)* **43,** 559 (1977).

172. J. Komatsu and S. Yoshikawa: *Rep. Quantum Electron. Meet. IECE Jpn.* **QE71−50** (1972).

173. A. N. Rubinov and V. A. Mostovnikov: *J. Appl. Spektrosk. (Engl. Transl.)* **7,** 223 (1967).

174. S. Mory, D. Leopold, R. Konig, P. Hoffman, and W. Fregin: *Exp. Tech. Phys.* **24,** 37 (1976).

175. W. E. K. Gibbs and H. A. Kellock: *IEEE J. Quantum Electron.* **QE−3,** 419 (1967).

176. F. G. Webster and W. C. McColgin: U.S. Patent No. 3,852,683 (1974).

177. G. A. Abakumov, A. P. Simonov, V. V. Fadeev, L. A. Kharitonov, and R. V. Khokhlov: *JETP Lett. (Engl. Transl.)* **9,** 9 (1969).

178. G. A. Abakumov, A. P. Simonov, V. V. Fadeev, M. A. Ka-symdganov, L. A. Kharitonov, and R. V. Khokhlov: *Opto-electronics (London)* **1,** 205 (1969).

179. M. Maeda, O. Uchino, E. Doi, K. Watanabe, and Y. Miyazoe: *IEEE J. Quantum Electron.* **QE−13,** 65 (1977).

180. D. G. Sutton and G. A. Capelle: *Appl. Phys. Lett.* **29,** 563 (1976).

181. B. Godard and O. de Witte: *Opt. Commun.* **19,** 325 (1976).

182. V. N. Lisitsyn, A. M. Razhev, and A. A. Chernenko: *Sov. J. Quantum Electron. (Engl. Transl.)* **8,** 244 (1978).

183. L. D. Ziegler and B. S. Hudson: *Opt. Commun.* **32,** 119 (1980).

184. P. R. Hammond, A. N. Fletcher, R. A. Henry, and R. L. Atkins: *Appl. Phys.* **8,** 311, 315 (1975); P. R. Hammond, A. N. Fletcher, D. E. Bliss, R. A. Henry, R. L. Atkins, and D. W. Moore: *Appl. Phys.* **9,**

67 (1976).

185. J. A. Myer, I. Itzkan, and E. Kierstead: *Nature (London)* **225**, 544 (1970).

186. T. Morrow and H. T. W. Price: *Opt. Commun.* **10**, 133 (1974).

187. O. R. Wood II, L. H. Szeto, and W. T. Silfvast: *J. Appl. Phys.* **48**, 1956 (1977).

188. V. S. Zuev, O. A. Logunov, Yu. V. Savinov, A. V. Startsev, and Yu. Yu. Stoilov: *Appl. Phys.* **17**, 321 (1978).

189. T. J. McKee, B. P. Stoicheff, and S. C. Wallace: *Opt. Lett.* **3**, 207 (1978).

190. T. J. McKee and D. J. James: *Can. J. Phys.* **57**, 1432 (1979).

191. K. L. Matheson and J. M. Thorne: *Appl. Phys. Lett.* **33**, 803 (1978).

192. K. Azuma, O. Nakagawa, Y. Segawa, Y. Aoyagi, and S. Namba: *Jpn. J. Appl. Phys.* **18**, 209 (1979).

193. T. F. Deutsch and M. Bass: *IEEE J. Quantum Electron.* **QE–5**, 261 (1969).

194. C. A. Turek and J. T. Yardley: *IEEE J. Quantum Electron.* **QE–7**, 102 (1971).

195. D. W. Fahey and L. D. Schearer: *IEEE J. Quantum Electron.* **QE–14**, 220 (1978).

196. W. Hüffer, R. Schieder, H. Telle, R. Raue, and W. Brinkwerth: *Opt. Commun.* **28**, 353 (1979).

197. H. Telle, U. Brinkmann, and R. Raue: *Opt. Commun.* **24**, 33 (1978).

198. W. Majewski and J. Krasinski: *Opt. Commun.* **18**, 255 (1976).

199. J. Kuhl, H. Telle, R. Schieder, and U. Brinkmann: *Opt. Commun.* **24**, 251 (1978).

200. I. M. Beterov, V. N. Ishchenko, B. Ya. Kogan, B. M. Krasovitskii, and A. A. Chernenko: *Sov. J. Quantum Electron. (Engl. Transl.)* **7**, 246 (1977).

201. A. J. Cox, G. W. Scott, and L. D. Talley: *Appl. Phys. Lett.* **31**, 389 (1977).

202. V. D. Kotsubanov, L. Ya. Malkes, Yu. V. Naboikin, L. A. Ogurtsova, A. P. Podgornyi, and F. S. Pokrovskaya: *Bull. Acad. Sci. USSR Phys. (Engl. Transl.)* Ser. **32**, 1357 (1968).

203. H. Telle, U. Brinkmann, and R. Raue: *Opt. Commun.* **24**, 248 (1978).

204. C. Rulliere, J. P. Morand, and J. Joussot-Dubien: *Opt. Commun.* **15**, 263 (1975).

205. E. Lill, S. Schneider, and F. Dörr: *Opt. Commun.* **20**, 223 (1977).

206. M. Lambropoulos: *Opt. Commun.* **15**, 35 (1975).

207. Yu. V. Naboikin, L. A. Ogurtsova, A. P. Podgornyi, and L. Ya. Malkes: *Sov. J. Quantum Electron (Engl. Transl.)* **8**, 457 (1978).

208. B. B. Snavely and O. G. Peterson: *IEEE J. Quantum Electron.* **QE–4**, 540 (1968).

209. V. I. Tomin, N. A. Nemkovich, and A. N. Rubinov: *Sov. J. Quantum Electron.* (*Engl. Transl.*) **8**, 567 (1978).
210. M. Takakusa and U. Itoh: *Opt. Commun.* **26**, 401 (1978).
211. M. Takakusa, U. Itoh, H. Anzai, H. Masuko, and T. Sato: *Jpn. J. Appl. Phys.* **17**, 1461 (1978).
212. U. Itoh, M. Takakusa, T. Moriya, and S. Saito: *Jpn. J. Appl. Phys.* **16**, 1059 (1977).
213. M. I. Dzyubenko, G. S. Vodotyka, V. V. Maslov, and V. M. Nikitchenko: *Opt. Spektrosk.* (*Engl. Transl.*) **39**, 310 (1975).
214. B. B. Snavely, O. G. Peterson, and R. F. Reithel: *Appl. Phys. Lett.* **11**, 275 (1967).
215. C. V. Shank, A. Dienes, A. M. Trozzolo, and J. A. Myer: *Appl. Phys. Lett.* **16**, 405 (1970).
216. S. A. Tuccio, K. H. Drexhage, and G. A. Reynolds: *Opt. Commun.* **7**, 248 (1973).
217. E. J. Schimitschek, J. A. Trias, P. R. Hammond. and R. L. Atkins: *Opt. Commun.* **11**, 352 (1974).
218. P. Crozet, B. S. Kirkiacharian, C. Soula, and Y. H. Meyer: *J. Chim. Phys. Phys. Chim. Biol.* **68**, 1388 (1971).
219. N. Ishibashi, T. Imasaka, T. Ogawa, M. Maeda, and Y. Miyazoe: *Chem. Lett.* **1974**, 1315 (1974); T. Imasaka, T. Ogawa, and N. Ishibashi: *Bull. Chem. Soc. Jpn.* **49**, 2687 (1976).
220. F. B. Dunning and R. F. Stebbings: *Opt. Commun.* **11**, 112 (1974).
221. K. Kato: *IEEE J. Quantum Electron.* **QE–11**, 373 (1975).
222. E. J. Schimitschek, J. A. Trias, P. R. Hammond, R. A. Henry, and R. L. Atkins: *Opt. Commun.* **16**, 313 (1976).
223. G. A. Reynolds and K. H. Drexhage: *Opt. Commun.* **13**, 222 (1975).
224. R. G. Morton, M. E. Mack, and I. Itzkan: *Appl. Opt.* **17**, 3268 (1978).
225. R. Srinivasan: *IEEE J. Quantum Electron.* **QE–5**, 552 (1969).
226. R. J. Gutfeld, B. Welber, and E. E. Tynan: *IEEE J. Quantum Electron.* **QE–6**, 532 (1970).
227. R. Wallenstein and H. Zacharias: *Opt. Commun.* **32**, 429 (1980).
228. O. S. Wolfbeis: *Monatsh. Chem.* **109**, 905 (1978).
229. M. R. Kagan, G. I. Farmer, and B. G. Huth: *Laser Focus* **4**, 26 (1968).
230. P. P. Sorokin and J. R. Lankard: *Phys. Rev.* **186**, 342 (1969).
231. C. M. Ferrar: *IEEE J. Quantum Electron.* **QE–5**, 550 (1969).
232. H. P. Broida and S. C. Haydon: *Appl. Phys. Lett.* **16**, 142 (1970).
233. J. Bunkenburg: *Rev. Sci. Instrum.* **43**, 1611 (1972).
234. E. J. Schimitschek, J. A. Trias, M. Taylor, and J. E. Celto: *IEEE J. Quantum Electron.* **QE–9**, 781 (1973).
235. C. B. Collins, K. N. Taylor, and F. W. Lee: *Opt. Commun.* **26**, 101 (1978).
236. J. A. Halstead and R. R. Reeves: *Opt. Commun.* **27**, 273 (1978).
237. J. C. Mialocq and P. Goujon: *Appl. Phys. Lett.* **33**, 819 (1978).

238. S. Saikan: *Appl. Phys.* **17**, 41 (1978).
239. J. C. Mialocq and P. Goujon: *Opt. Commun.* **24**, 255 (1978).
240. G. A. Abakumov, M. M. Mestechkin, V. N. Poltavets, and A. P. Simonov: *Sov. J. Quantum Electron.* (*Engl. Transl.*) **8**, 1115 (1978).
241. A. Dienes, C. V. Shank, and R. L. Kohn: *IEEE J. Quantum Electron.* **QE–9**, 833 (1973).
242. W. Hüffer, R. Schieder, H. Telle, R. Raue, and W. Brinkwerth: *Opt. Commun.* **33**, 85 (1980).
243. W. Zapka and U. Brackmann: *Appl. Phys.* **20**, 283 (1979).
244. N. A. Borisevich, V. A. Povedailo, and V. A. Tolkachev: *Opt. Commun.* **33**, 203 (1980).
245. B. Steyer and F. P. Schäfer: *Appl. Phys.* **7**, 113 (1975).
246. B. Steyer and F. P. Schäfer: *Opt. Commun.* **10**, 219 (1974).
247. P. W. Smith, P. F. Liao, C. V. Shank, T. K. Gustafson, D. Lin, and P. J. Maloney: *Appl. Phys. Lett.* **25**, 144 (1974).
248. G. Marowsky, R. Cordray, F. K. Tittel, W. L. Wilson, and C. B. Collins: *Appl. Phys. Lett.* **33**, 59 (1978).
249. A. N. Fletcher: Naval Weapons Center (NWC) **TP 5768** (1975).
250. C. Rullière and J. Joussot-Dubien: *Opt. Commun.* **24**, 38 (1978).
251. C. Rullière, J. P. Morand, and O. de Witte: *Opt. Commun.* **20**, 339 (1977).
252. D. Cotter: *Opt. Commun.* **31**, 397 (1979).
253. L. Ducasse: Doctoral Thesis, Bordeaux Univ., France, 1976.
254. C. Rullière and J.-C. Rayez: *Appl. Phys.* **11**, 377 (1976).
255. M. E. Mack: *Appl. Phys. Lett.* **19**, 108 (1971).
256. L. A. Lee and R. A. Robb: *IEEE J. Quantum Electron.* **QE–16**, 777 (1980).
257. F. P. Schäfer, Zs. Bor, W. Lüttke, and B. Liphardt: *Chem. Phys. Lett.* **56**, 455 (1978).
258. B. S. Neporent and V. B. Shilov: *Opt. Spektrosk.* **30**, 576 (1971).
259. A. V. Aristov and V. A. Kuzin: *Opt. Spektrosk.* (*Engl. Transl.*) **32**, 57 (1971).
260. L. G. Pikulik, V. A. Yakovenko, and A. D. Das'ko: *Zh. Prikl. Spectrosk.* **23**, 493 (1975).
261. V. S. Smirnov and N. G. Bakhshiev: *Opt. Spektrosk.* (*Engl. Transl.*) **43**, 697 (1977).
262. Yu. E. Zabiyakin, V. S. Smirnov, and N. G. Bakhshiev: *Opt. Spektrosk.* (*Engl. Transl.*) **35**, 675 (1973).
263. M. Kleinerman and M. Dabrowski: *Opt. Commun.* **26**, 81 (1978).
264. O. S. Wolfbeis, W. Rapp, and E. Lippert: *Monatsh. Chem.* **109**, 899 (1978).
265. A. N. Fletcher, D. A. Fine, and D. E. Bliss: *Appl. Phys.* **12**, 39 (1977).

266. A. N. Fletcher: *Appl. Phys.* **12**, 327 (1977).
267. A. N. Fletcher: *Appl. Phys.* **14**, 295 (1977).
268. A. N. Fletcher: *Appl. Phys.* **16**, 93 (1978).
269. A. N. Fletcher and D. E. Bliss: *Appl. Phys.* **16**, 289 (1978).
270. I. B. Berlman: "Handbook of Fluorescence Spectra of Aromatic Molecules." Academic Press, New York, 1971.
271. T. Sakurai: *Laser Kenkyu* **7**, 125 (1979).
272. P. W. Smith, P. F. Liao, and P. J. Maloney: *IEEE J. Quantum Electron.* **QE–12**, 539 (1976).
273. B. H. Soffer and B. B. McFarland: *Appl. Phys. Lett.* **10**, 266 (1967).
274. S. L. Shapiro (ed.): "Ultrashort Light Pulses." Springer-Verlag, Berlin, 1977.
275. M. Bass, T. F. Deutsch, and M. J. Weber: in "Lasers" (A. K. Levine and A. J. DeMaria, eds.), Vol. 3. Dekker, New York, 1971.
276. F. P. Schäfer: "Laser Handbook" (F. T. Arecchi and E. O. Schulz-Dubois, eds.). North Holland, Amsterdam, 1972.
277. J. M. Kauffman: *Appl. Opt.* **19**, 3431 (1980).
278. G. Marowsky: *IEEE J. Quantum Electron.* **QE–16**, 49 (1980).
279. H. W. Furumoto and H. L. Ceccon: *Appl. Opt.* **8**, 1613 (1969).
280. C. M. Ferrar: *Rev. Sci. Instrum.* **40**, 1436 (1969).
281. T. Okada, K. Fujiwara, M. Maeda, and Y. Miyazoe: *Appl. Phys.* **15**, 191 (1978).
282. M. E. Mack: *Appl. Opt.* **13**, 46 (1974).
283. C. K. Rhodes (ed.): "Excimer Lasers." Springer-Verlag, Berlin, 1978.
284. O. G. Peterson, J. P. Webb, and W. C. McColgin: *J. Appl. Phys.* **42**, 1917 (1971).
285. T. W. Hänsch: *Appl. Opt.* **11**, 895 (1972).
286. I. Shoshan, N. N. Danon, and U. P. Oppenheim: *J. Appl. Phys.* **48**, 4495 (1977).
287. M. G. Littman and H. J. Metcalf: *Appl. Opt.* **17**, 2224 (1978).
288. H. Kogelnik and C. V. Shank: *Appl. Phys. Lett.* **18**, 152 (1971).
289. C. V. Shank, J. E. Bjorkholm, and H. Kogelnik: *Appl. Phys. Lett.* **18**, 395 (1971).
290. W. H. Glenn, M. J. Brienza, and A. J. DeMaria: *Appl. Phys. Lett.* **12**, 54 (1968).
291. L. J. E. Hofer, R. J. Grabenstetter, and E. O. Wiig: *J. Am. Chem. Soc.* **72**, 203 (1950).
292. "Catalogue of Nippon Kanko Shikiso Kenkyusho" (1-2-3 Shimo-Ishii, Okayama 700, Japan).
293. Catalogue of Eastman Organic Chemicals" (Eastman Kodak Company, Ltd., Rochester, New York 14650).

294. P. K. Runge and R. Rosenberg: *IEEE J. Quantum Electron.* **QE-8**, 910 (1972).

295. P. Mazzinghi, P. Burlamacchi, M. Matera, H. F. Ranea-Sandoval, R. Salimbeni, and U. Vanni: *IEEE J. Quantum Electron.* **QE-17**, 2245 (1981).

296. J. R. Heldt, J. Szczepański, and J. Heldt: *Opt. Commun.* **39**, 325 (1981).

297. E. G. Marason: *Opt. Commun.* **37**, 56 (1981).

298. P. E. Jessop and A. Szabo: *IEEE J. Quantum Electron.* **QE-16**, 812 (1980).

299. B. Liphardt, B. Liphardt, and W. Lüttke: *Opt. Commun.* **38**, 207 (1981).

300. O. V. Przhonskaya, I. P. Il'chishin, E. A. Tikhonov, and Yu. L. Slominskiĭ: *Sov. J. Quantum Electron.* (*Engl. Transl.*) **9**, 16 (1979).

301. M. A. Al'perovich, G. G. Dyadyusha, O. V. Przhonskaya, T. N. Smirnova, Yu. L. Slominskiĭ, E. A. Tikhonov, A. I. Tolmachev, V. S. Tyurin, and M. T. Shpak: *Sov. J. Quantum Electron.* (*Engl. Transl.*) **9**, 725 (1979).

302. F. G. Zhang and F. P. Schäfer: *Appl. Phys.* **B26**, 211 (1981).

303. T. F. Johnston, Jr., R. H. Brady, and W. Proffitt: *Appl. Opt.* **21**, 2307 (1982).

304. E. G. Marason: *Opt. Commun.* **40**, 212 (1982).

305. W. G. Divens and S. M. Jarrett: *Rev. Sci. Instrum.* **53**, 1363 (1982).

306. R. S. Taylor and P. B. Corkum: *Appl. Phys.* **B26**, 31 (1981).

307. W. Sibbett and J. R. Taylor: *Opt. Commun.* **44**, 121 (1982).

308. W. Sibbett and J. R. Taylor: *Opt. Commun.* **43**, 50 (1982).

309. T. Varghese: *Opt. Commun.* **44**, 353 (1983).

310. G. White and J. G. Pruett: *Opt. Lett* **6**, 473 (1981).

311. D. J. Eilenberger, E. D. Isaacs, and G. D. Aumiller: *Opt. Commun.* **44**, 350 (1983).

312. G. D. Aumiller: *Opt. Commun.* **41**, 115 (1982).

313. R. K. Jain: *Appl. Phys. Lett.* **40**, 295 (1982).

314. M. Sanchez Gomez and J. M. Guerra Perez: *Opt. Commun.* **40**, 144 (1981).

315. K. Kato: *J. Quantum Electron.* **16**, 1017 (1980).

316. J. Hoffnagle, L. Ph. Roesch, N. Schlumpf, and A. Weis: *Opt. Commun.* **42**, 267 (1982).

317. J. Hoffnagle, L. Ph. Roesch, N. Schlumpf, A. Weis, and K. Kato: *Opt. Commun.* **44**, 53 (1982).

Wavelength Index

The tunable range of dye lasers is divided into 30 regions, and all the dye code numbers (#M) whose lasing wavelengths are included in the given region are described. The widest tunable range recorded in each table is taken.

Wavelength (nm)	Code number
300–325	#M206, 208
325–350	#M206, 208, 209, 211, 435, 439, 440, 441, 442, 448, 449
350–375	#M206, 208, 209, 210, 211, 212*, 269, 411, 418, 430, 439, 443, 444, 445, 446, 450, 451, 455, 456, #M457, 459, 462, 463, 464, 465, 467, 472
375–400	#M209, 210, 212*, 216, 217, 218*, 221, 222, 223, 224, 229, 269, 271, 272, 273, 274, 281, 283, 400, #M405, 408, 411, 413, 416, 417, 418, 426, 430, 432, 438, 439, 455, 456, 457, 458, 459, 460, 461, #M463, 465, 466, 467, 468, 469, 470, 472, 488, 534
400–425	#M133, 171, 172, 173, 174, 192, 193, 194, 201, 202, 207, 210, 212*, 213, 215, 217, 218*, 219, 225, #M226, 227, 228, 229, 230, 231, 232, 233, 234, 235, 236, 237*, 238, 239, 240, 241, 242, 243, 244 #M245, 246, 247, 248, 249, 252, 253, 254, 255, 257, 258, 259, 260*, 262, 263, 264, 266, 267, 268, #M270, 271, 272, 278, 280, 281, 283, 284, 286, 292, 294, 296, 300, 301, 311*, 313, 315, 362, 364, #M365, 372, 378, 381, 383, 384, 386*, 387, 388, 389, 390, 392, 394, 396, 397, 401, 406, 412, 413, #M416, 417, 419, 420, 421, 423, 426, 427, 432, 434, 436, 438, 447, 452, 453, 454, 455, 458, 465, #M468, 469, 471, 532, 534, 535, 536

550–575	#M86, 87, 88*, 90, 94*, 95, 97*, 100, 102, 112*, 113, 114*, 115, 117, 120, 121, 130, 159, 161, 195, #M196, 198, 199, 200, 276, 281, 319, 327, 334*, 336*, 345, 353, 481, 485, 486, 500, 507, 511, 533
575–600	#M84, 85, 86, 87, 88*, 89, 90, 92, 93, 94*, 95, 96, 97*, 100, 101, 103, 104, 106, 108, 109, 110, #M111, 112*, 114*, 116*, 121, 132, 141, 195, 196, 199, 276, 334*, 353, 483, 484, 486
600–625	#M1, 3, 17, 78*, 84, 85, 86, 87, 88*, 89, 90*, 91, 92*, 93, 94*, 95, 97*, 98, 99, 107, 109*, 110*, 132, 140, 141, 142, 149, 158, 160, 162, 276, 483, 486, 508, 521, 525, 526, 527
625–650	#M1, 17, 78*, 85, 90*, 92*, 93, 94*, 98, 109*, 110*, 135, 137, 140, 141, 150, 156, 157, 509, 519
650–675	#M10, 17, 78*, 85, 90*, 92*, 94*, 109*, 110*, 134, 137, 138, 140*, 141, 143, 151, 156, 157, 166, 498
675–700	#M10, 17, 78*, 80, 81, 82, 83, 90*, 92*, 109*, 110*, 122, 134, 136*, 138, 139*, 140*, 141, 143, 146, 153, 154, 166*, 167
700–725	#M4, 10*, 11, 14, 15, 16, 18, 41, 43, 44, 75, 78*, 82, 109*, 122, 134, 136*, 138, 139*, 140, 141, #M143, 153, 154, 155, 166*, 167*
725–750	#M5, 6, 10*, 11, 13, 18, 20, 21, 24, 38, 41, 43*, 44, 75, 82, 134, 136*, 139*, 141, 144*, 153, 154, 166*, 167*
750–755	#M4, 6, 10*, 11, 14, 15, 20, 22, 24, 30, 39, 41, 43*, 44*, 64, 79, 80, 82, 123, 124, 127, 134, #M136*, 139*, 144*, 163, 167*
775–800	#M12, 14, 15, 20, 23, 28, 29, 30, 40, 43*, 44*, 45, 46, 64, 74, 76, 136*, 139*, 144*, 152, 164, 165, 167*
800–850	#M6, 20, 22, 28, 29*, 32, 34, 35, 36, 37, 40, 42, 43*, 44*, 46*, 48, 49, 63*, 64, 65, 76, 125, 126, 136*, 144*, 145, 146, 147, 148, 152, 165, 167*
850–900	#M20, 25, 29*, 31, 32, 33, 34, 35, 36, 37, 42, 43*, 44*, 46*, 47*, 49, 50, 52, 53*, 54, 56*, 57, 58*, #M59, 60, 63*, 79, 144*, 145
900–950	#M20, 25, 32, 35, 46*, 47*, 49, 50, 53*, 55, 56*, 58*, 60*, 63, 66*, 67, 77, 144*
950–1000	#M20, 35, 47*, 49, 50, 51, 53*, 56*, 58*, 60*, 63, 66*
1000–1050	#M20, 51, 53*, 56, 58*, 60*, 66*, 68, 71

1050–1100	#M51, 58*, 66*, 68, 69, 71, 72, 73
1100–1150	#M51, 68, 69, 70, 71, 72, 73
1150–1200	#M69, 70, 71, 73
1200–1250	#M70, 73
1250–1300	#M70

*Indicates that the CW operation is possible.

Compound Index

A

B

I

IR-107, #M77; IR-109, #M54; IR-123, #M64; IR-125, #M49;
 IR-132, #M60; IR-134, #M59; IR-135; #M65; IR-136,
 #M61; IR-137, #M53; IR-139, #M57; IR-140, #M56;
 IR-141, #M55; IR-143, #M58; IR-144, #M63; IR-145,
 #M62; IR-166, #M31
Isoquinoline red   #M158

K

Kiton red 620, #M92; kiton red S, #M92

L

Lachs   #M275
LD390, #M408; LD423, #M397; LD425, #M378; LD466,
 #M329; LD473, #M399; LD490, #M351; LD690,
 #M166; LD700, #M167
Leukophor B, #M232; Leukophor DC, #M265
Lissamine rhodamine B-200   #M93
Lucigenin   #M132

M

Magnesium phthalocyanine   #M80
Merocyanine B   #M76
Metal free phthalocyanine   #M79
1-(7-Methoxy-2H-2-oxo-1-benzopyran-3-yl)-3-methyl-   #M299
 1H-1,2,3-triazolium methylsulfate
N-[4-(7-Methoxy-2H-2-oxo-1-benzopyran-3-yl)phenyl]-   #M298
 trimethylammonium methylsulfate
7-Methoxy-3-carbethoxycoumarin   #M300
2′-Methoxy-1,4-distyrylbenzene   #M247
3′-Methoxy-1,4-distyrylbenzene   #M248
4′-Methoxy-1,4-distyrylbenzene   #M249
4-Methoxy-αNPD   #M460
6-Methoxy umbelliferone   #M293
N-Methylacridinium perchlorate   #M130
7-Methylamino-4,6-dimethylcoumarin   #M315
9-Methylanthracene   #M174
4-Methyl-7-bis(3-sulfopropyl)aminocoumarin disodium salt   #M339
Methyl DOTC   #M43
Methylene blue   #M146

N

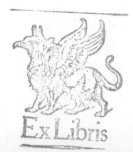